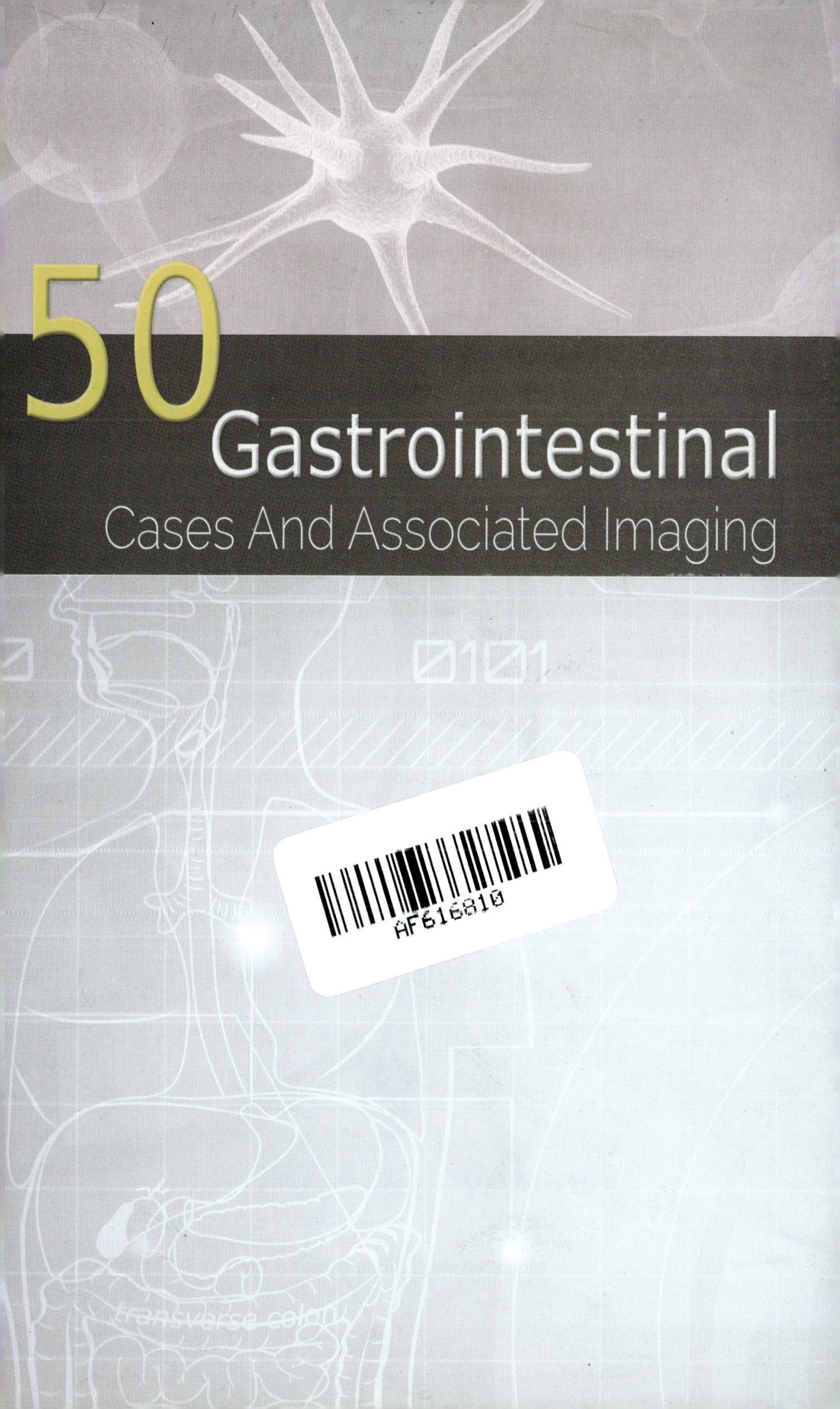

50 Gastrointestinal
Cases And Associated Imaging

50 Gastrointestinal Cases and Associated imaging

by

Abdullah A. Shaikh/ Syed M. Hussain/ David J. Desilets/ Tara M. Catazano

Medical knowledge is constantly changing. As new information becomes available, changes in treatment, procedures, equipment and the use of drugs become necessary. The editors, contributors and the publishers have, as far as it is possible, taken care to ensure that the information given in this text is accurate and up-to-date. However, readers are strongly advised to confirm that the information, especially with regard to drug usage, complies with the latest legislation and standards of practice. Neither the publisher nor the authors assume any responsibility for any loss or injury and/or damage to person or property arising out of or related to any use of the material contained in this handbook.

This **SAARC** edition is published by Paramount Books
in arrangement with tfm Publishing Limited - UK

ISBN: 978-969-637-229-5

Printed in Pakistan 2017

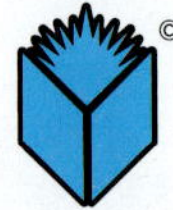

Paramount Books (Pvt) Ltd.

152/O, Block-2, P.E.C.H.S., Karachi-75400. Tel: 34310030
Fax: 34553772, E-mail: info@paramountbooks.com.pk
Website: www.paramountbooks.com.pk

Contents

Foreword

This book is a unique collaborative effort from physicians trained in medicine, gastroenterology, and radiology. It is the brainchild of two former internal medicine residents: Abdullah Shaikh and Syed Hussain. Abdullah is currently a radiology resident with an interest in gastrointestinal imaging, and Syed is a GI fellow specializing in hepatobiliary disease. This book would not have been possible without the mentorship of David Desilets, who has kept a stack of interesting endoscopic images and cases over several decades, and provided expert guidance and oversight. Tara Catanzano, a radiologist with a multispecialty imaging background, provided expertise and was an integral part of this project. Incidentally, three of the authors are graduates of the Royal College of Surgeons in Ireland, and have incorporated aspects of their Irish education into this book.

We hope that you, the reader, will fall in love with GI imaging as we have done. Perhaps it will spark your interest in GI diseases. Each individual case stands alone, requires no other chapter to support it, and provides a few clinical pearls that may come in handy on rounds. The book will possibly help you in caring for your patients, or will be recalled with a smile when you are sitting for board exams. The cases are best read one at a time, in your spare time, so that a few clinical pearls will be absorbed once in a while. It is not a textbook or reference book. We hope you will learn that the approach to GI illnesses involves a synthesis of all the available data: historical, physical, radiographic, laboratory, and endoscopic. Putting this information together to solve the patient's puzzle is what's so fun about medicine in general, and gastroenterology in particular.

Abdullah A. Shaikh MD
Department of Medicine and Radiology Baystate Medical Center/Tufts University Springfield, Massachusetts, USA

Syed M. Hussain MD MRCS
Department of Medicine University of Cincinnati Cincinnati, Ohio, USA

David J. Desilets MD PhD
Department of Medicine Baystate Medical Center/Tufts University Springfield, Massachusetts, USA

Tara M. Catanzano MD
Department of Radiology Baystate Medical Center/Tufts University Springfield, Massachusetts, USA

Abbreviations

ABD	abdomen
ABG	arterial blood gas
ALT	alanine transaminase
AMA	anti-mitochondrial antibody
ANA	anti-nuclear antibody
ASA	American Society of Anesthesiologists
AST	aspartate transaminase
bHCG	β-human chorionic gonadotrophin
BP	blood pressure
BUN	blood urea nitrogen
CA 19.9	carbohydrate antigen 19.9
CBC	complete blood count
CHEM-6	chemistry 6
CHEM-7	chemistry 7
CK-MB	creatine kinase-MB
Cl	chloride
COPD	chronic obstructive pulmonary disease
CPR	cardiopulmonary resuscitation
CRP	C-reactive protein
CT	computed tomography
CVS	cardiovascular
DEXA	dual-energy X-ray absorptiometry
EGD	esophagogastroduodenoscopy
EKG	electrocardiogram
ERCP	endoscopic retrograde cholangiopancreatography
ESR	erythrocyte sedimentation rate
EXT	extremities
GEN	general
GGT	γ-glutamyl transferase
GI	gastrointestinal
H+N	head and neck
HAART	highly active antiretroviral therapy
HbA1c	glycated hemoglobin
HEENT	head, eyes, ears, nose, throat
HIDA	hepatobiliary iminodiacetic acid
HIV	human immunodeficiency virus
HR	heart rate
Ig	immunoglobulin
INR	international normalized ratio
IV	intravenous
K	potassium
LDH	lactate dehydrogenase
LFT	liver function test
MCV	mean corpuscular volume
MRCP	magnetic resonance cholangiopancreatography
MRI	magnetic resonance imaging
MSK	musculoskeletal
Na	sodium
NSAID	non-steroidal anti-inflammatory drug
p-ANCA	perinuclear anti-neutrophil cytoplasmic antibodies
PET	positron emission tomography
RA	room air
RBC	red blood cell
RESP	respiratory
TSH	thyroid-stimulating hormone
WBC	white blood cell

Case 1

A 44-year-old woman presents to the emergency room with right upper quadrant pain. The pain began about 20 minutes after eating dinner. It is described as a "shooting pain" that is constant, radiates to her back, and is 6/10 in intensity. The pain is worse on deep inspiration, and a tablet of oxycodone offers some relief. She denies nausea or vomiting. Her bowel movements are regular. She has never had this pain before.

What is your differential diagnosis?

The differential diagnosis includes cholelithiasis, acute cholecystitis, pancreatitis, gastritis, peptic ulcer disease, gastric volvulus, and intussusception.

Physical examination

Vitals Afebrile, HR 88 bpm, BP 130/78mmHg, oxygen saturation 99% o n RA.

GEN No distress.

HEENT No scleral icterus.

CVS Normal S1, S2. No murmurs, rubs, or gallops.

RESP Clear to auscultation.

ABD Soft and non-tender. No rigidity, guarding, or rebound tenderness. Bowel sounds are normal. Rectal examination reveals an empty vault.

EXT No edema.

Does this narrow your differential diagnosis?

Yes. Volvulus and intussusception can be removed from the differential diagnosis, as bowel sounds are altered in these clinical settings.

What blood test(s) will you order?

LFTs	AST	267 units/L
	ALT	285 units/L
	Alkaline phosphatase	262 units/L
	Total bilirubin	3.6mg/dL

What is the pattern of the elevated LFTs?

Elevated LFTs usually suggest either a hepatocellular process or an obstructive (or cholestatic) process. A cholestatic process presents with elevated alkaline phosphatase and elevated total bilirubin levels. With the passage of a gallstone through the common bile duct, ALT may be the first measure to appear abnormal.

What other blood tests will you order?

CBC, CHEM-7, and bHCG.

All are within normal limits.

What imaging test will you order?

Your differential diagnosis already includes gallbladder pathology. Therefore, an ultrasound is the most important imaging test. The probe is placed over the ninth rib costal margin in the right mid-clavicular line. You see the image shown in Figure 1.

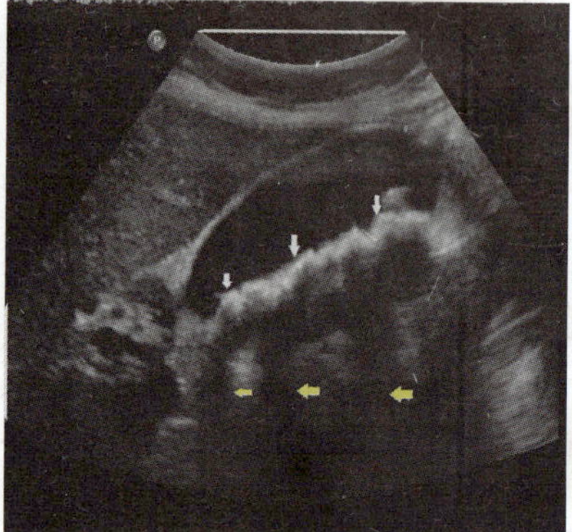

Figure 1.

Describe what you see and read on

The ultrasound shows a gallbladder in the sagittal view. Gallstones (white arrows) cast dark shadows (yellow arrows) on ultrasound. Changing the patient's position demonstrates the stones are mobile. This image does not show a thickened gallbladder wall, or a black rim around the gallbladder wall suggesting fluid (pericholecystic fluid). The patient's Murphy's sign was negative on physical examination.

By now you have admitted the patient, kept her nil by mouth, started IV fluids, and called for a surgical consultation. Later you receive the radiology report and notice the patient's common bile duct is 8mm.

What is your initial diagnosis, and how will you proceed?

The diameter of the common bile duct, measured in millimeters, should be less than or equal to the patient's age in decades. So for this 44-year-old patient, who is in her fifth decade, it should be 5mm or less. An 8mm bile duct is suggestive, but not diagnostic, of at least some degree of biliary obstruction, and liver enzymes elevated in an obstructive pattern support this diagnosis. Given the numerous gallstones seen on ultrasound, a working diagnosis of choledocholithiasis — common duct stone(s) — is reasonable.

The next step is to obtain a GI consultation for a possible ERCP. This is arranged for the next day. The image shown in Figure 2 is obtained during the procedure.

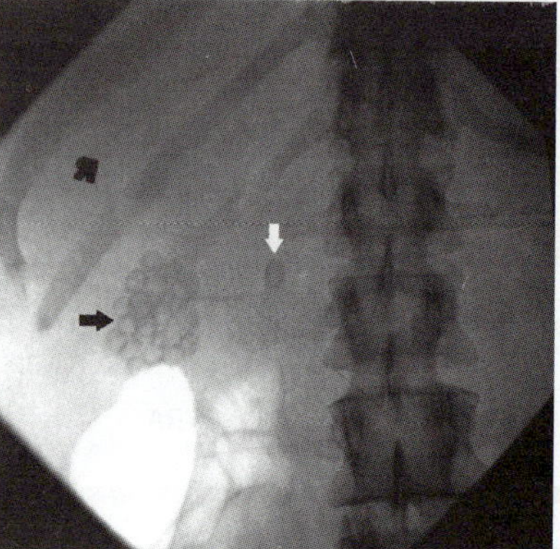

Figure 2.

Describe what you see and read on

A fluoroscopic scout view of the right upper quadrant is obtained prior to the endoscopic procedure. Numerous stones are present in the gallbladder (black arrow). In addition, a solitary stone is seen outside the expected location of the gallbladder (white arrow), suggesting a stone in the biliary tree. A fluoroscopic image is obtained during the ERCP (Figure 3).

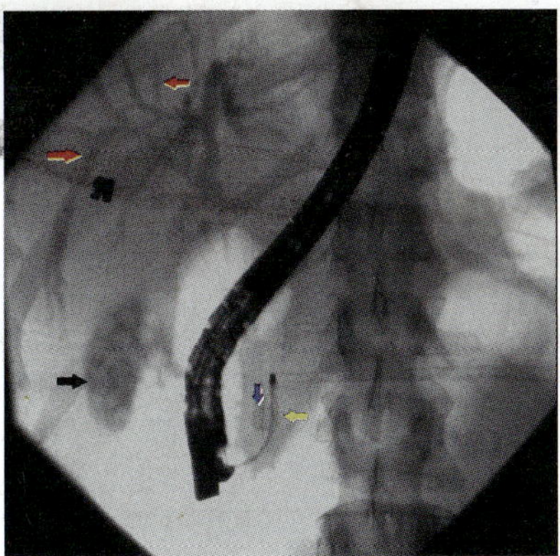

Figure 3.

Describe what you see and read on

This fluoroscopic image shows that the gallbladder (black arrow) and intrahepatic biliary ducts (red arrows) have been opacified with contrast. There is air in the common bile duct after biliary sphincterotomy, and a Dormia basket (yellow arrow) has engaged the stone (blue arrow) and is being used for its extraction.

A stone that was not seen on ultrasound was obstructing the common bile duct. This also explains why the patient had elevated LFTs, as the stone was causing biliary obstruction.

Overnight, the patient's laboratory results improved. She remained pain-free and was discharged with a plan to have a laparoscopic cholecystectomy at a later date.

Clinical pearl

- Only two-thirds of common duct stones are seen on ultrasound when the common bile duct is less than 10mm. In this case the ultrasound did not show the stone in the duct, but there was a high clinical suspicion based on clinical history, elevated LFTs, and the slightly dilated common bile duct at 8mm.

Impress your attending

What are gallstones made from?

Most gallstones (approximately 85%) are composed of cholesterol salts. The remaining stones are composed of pigment salts (calcium bilirubinate) and so are calcified and radiolucent. A small percentage combine both types. Factors that influence the likelihood of calcium bilirubinate stones include any process causing increased hemolysis or high red blood cell turnover, such as sickle-cell anemia, hereditary spherocytosis, thalassemia, and hypersplenism.

Case 2

A 47-year-old woman presents to the emergency room with increasing weakness over the past few months. Most of her time is spent in bed, and she feels no desire to do anything. When questioned very closely, she admits to intermittent vomiting, without hematemesis. She is not sure what brings on the vomiting. She describes some vague intermittent discomfort in the hypochondrium that radiates to her back when she eats. The patient has a decreased appetite and feels nauseated much of the time. She has lost about 20 lbs (9.1kg) over the past 3 months. She describes dyspnea on exertion. The patient recently lost a member of her family from stroke. Her stools are brown. She takes no NSAIDs or steroids. Her only medication is folic acid. She is known to have a uterine fibroid.

What is your differential diagnosis?

The differential diagnosis includes dyspepsia, peptic ulcer disease, malignancy, occult GI bleed, and depression.

Physical examination

Vitals Afebrile, HR 92 bpm, BP 110/74mmHg, oxygen saturation 98% on RA.

GEN Weak and cachectic-appearing.

Hands Pale palmar creases.

HEENT No scleral icterus. Pale conjunctivae.

CVS Normal S1, S2. Grade I systolic flow murmur. No rubs or gallops.

RESP Clear to auscultation.

ABD Soft and non-tender. A palpable 4-5cm mass is present in the suprapubic region. No rigidity, guarding, or rebound tenderness. Bowel sounds are normal. Rectal examination reveals brown stool (stool occult-positive).

EXT No edema.

What diagnosis does the physical examination suggest?

The diagnosis suggests anemia with possible underlying malignancy. The presence of blood in the stool suggests a gastric, colonic, or small-bowel lesion, and the palpable mass suggests malignancy.

What blood test(s) will you order?

CBC	**WBC**	10 x 10^3/μL
	Hemoglobin	3.7g/dL
	Hematocrit	12.7%
	Platelets	665 x 10^3/ μL
ESR		88mm/h

What other blood tests will you order?

CHEM-7, LFTs, and lipase.

All are within normal limits.

The patient is profoundly anemic and has abdominal pain. She also has a palpable mass and a prior CT scan confirming a very large uterus. Your first priority is to admit the patient, keep her nil by mouth, and obtain consent for a blood transfusion.

The next morning, the patient's hemoglobin level is up to 9g/dL and her hematocrit is at 30%. It is now time to determine why they were so low. She already has findings to explain why she might be losing blood. Further history confirms heavy menses, likely caused by her fibroid tumor. The palpable mass is probably a large fibroid (which is a benign mass). The anemia could explain the lethargy, but not the abdominal pain and weight loss.

What imaging test will you order?

You decide to order an upper GI study. The results are shown in Figure 4.

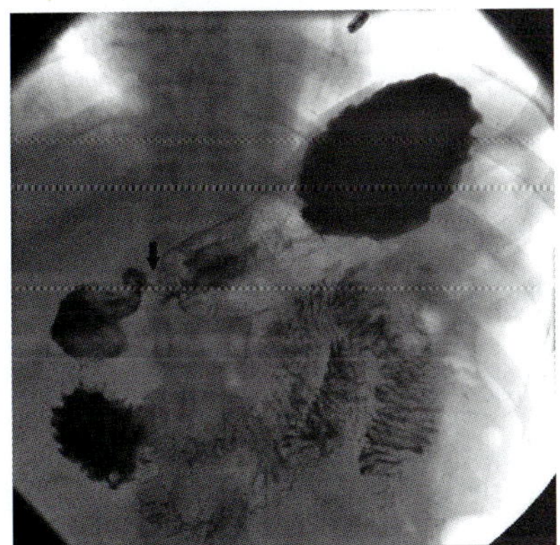

Figure 4.

Describe what you see and read on

Figure 4 shows an anterior view of the upper GI tract. The proximal stomach is adequately distended and unremarkable in appearance. The distal aspect of the stomach, including the pylorus and the proximal duodenum, is irregular in contour (black arrow) with loss of the normal mucosal pattern. The distal duodenum appears normal.

Given this image and the patient's presenting history, what are you concerned about?

You should be most concerned about gastric cancer, lymphoma, or peptic ulcer disease. The next step is to obtain a GI consultation requesting an EGD. The procedure results in the image shown in Figure 5.

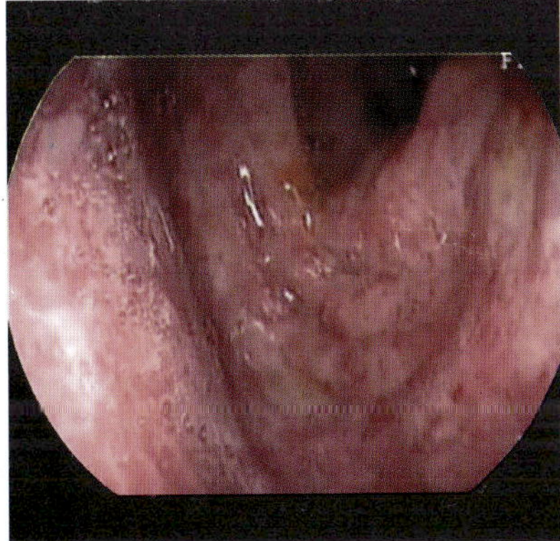

Figure 5.

Describe what you see and read on

The EGD shows erythema, edema, and multiple erosions of the antrum and duodenal bulb consistent with marked antral gastritis and bulbar duodenitis. Biopsies reveal *Helicobacter pylori*. The patient is treated with a proton-pump inhibitor and antibiotics for 2 weeks, and her pain gradually resolves. A test of cure is performed 8 weeks later with a urea breath test, which is negative.

The patient's anemia does not account for her other symptoms, as discussed earlier. A psychiatric evaluation is undertaken and the patient is found to be severely depressed. She is discharged to a psychiatry unit with oral iron therapy, proton-pump inhibitors, a bowel regimen, and follow-up with her obstetrician/gynecologist for consideration for hysterectomy or uterine embolization.

Clinical pearl

- Many regimens are available to treat *H. pylori.* You should remember the most generic version as it is the most affordable for patients:
  - a proton-pump inhibitor twice daily + clarithromycin 500mg twice daily + amoxicillin 1g twice daily for 10-14 days.

Impress you attending

What two reasons might explain this patient's increased platelets?

- Reactive thrombocytosis.
- Folic acid intake.

In iron-deficiency anemia, platelet counts can increase because of upregulated bone marrow. An increased platelet level will often be seen in women who are taking folic acid or prenatal vitamins.

Case 3

A 64-year-old woman presents at the clinic for a routine check-up. When she sees you in the examination room, she is delighted to hear she has lost 20 lbs. On further questioning she says she has become more fatigued and has not been able to keep up with her friends while doing aerobics, and often becoming "winded." She has no chest or abdominal pain. There have been no changes in the patient's appetite or in her bowel pattern or the caliber of the stools. The patient has yearly mammograms, which have all been normal. Her last colonoscopy was 9 years ago and showed a hyperplastic polyp. Her weight loss has been unintentional.

What is your differential diagnosis?

The differential diagnosis includes dyspepsia, peptic ulcer disease, malignancy, occult GI bleeding, and depression.

Physical examination

Vitals	Afebrile, HR 92 bpm, BP 110/74mmHg, oxygen saturation 98% on RA.
GEN	No obvious distress.
Hands	Clubbing. Pale palmar creases.
H+N	No scleral icterus.
CVS	Normal S1, S2. No murmurs, rubs, or gallops.
RESP	Clear to auscultation.
ABD	Soft and non-tender. No rigidity, guarding, or rebound tenderness. Palpable fullness in the left lower quadrant. Bowel sounds are present. Rectal examination reveals brown stool (stool occult-positive).
EXT	No edema.

What one blood test will you order?

CBC	WBC	10 x $10^3/\mu L$
	Hemoglobin	8.8g/dL
	Hematocrit	24.3%
	Platelets	421 x $10^3/\mu L$

What other blood tests will you order?

CHEM-7.

All are within normal limits.

What imaging test will you order?

A CT scan of the abdomen and pelvis with oral an d IV contrast. The image shown in Figure 6 is obtained.

Describe what you see and read on

This is a single coronal view of the abdomen. Circumferential narrowing of the ascending colon can be seen in the right lower quadrant, with areas of shouldering above and below the narrowing consistent with an 'apple-core' lesion (arrow). The remainder

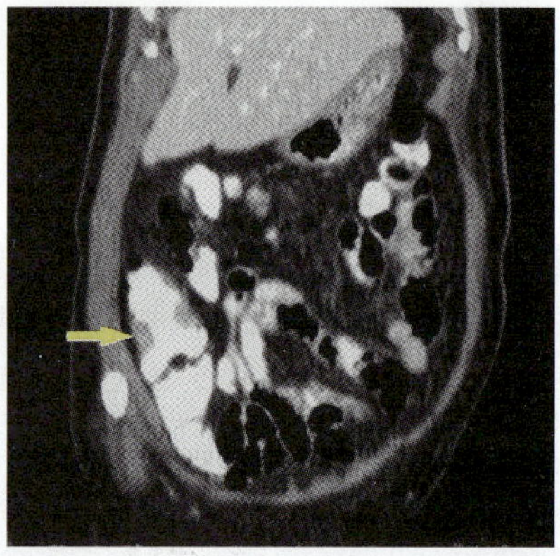

Figure 6.

of the visualized bowel wall does not demonstrate wall thickening. There is no free fluid or adenopathy. No liver lesions are present.

What is the next step?

The results are discussed and a referral to the GI consultant is made. The patient is scheduled for a colonoscopy within a couple of days. The colonoscopy results are shown in Figure 7.

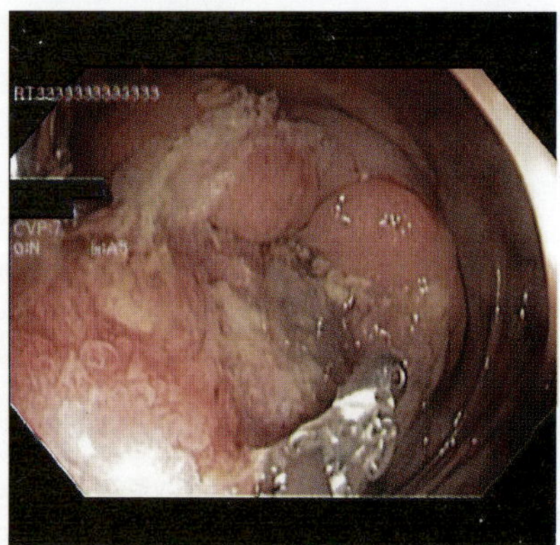

Figure 7.

Describe what you see and read on

The image obtained during colonoscopy shows a large fungating cecal mass. Biopsies of this cecal lesion were taken during the colonoscopy, and these returned a diagnosis of adenocarcinoma. The next step would be to refer the patient to surgery for a right hemicolectomy, and to medical oncology for further evaluation and follow-up.

Clinical pearl

- Most adenocarcinomas of the colon are believed to arise from adenomatous polyps. We know from surveillance barium enemas in patients who refuse surgery or are poor surgical candidates that the adenoma-to-carcinoma sequence takes approximately 10 years. If an adenoma is found on colonoscopy, the next colonoscopy is usually recommended for 5 years later (unless the polyp is large or three or more adenomas are found). The fact that this patient's colonoscopy 9 years previously failed to protect her from developing colon cancer could be for several reasons:
  - the cancer is on the right side. It could be the colonoscopy was not completed;
  - this lesion would probably have been very small 9 years ago, if present at all. A small lesion such as this can easily be missed, especially if the preparation is poor;
  - finally, this could be a fast-growing adenocarcinoma, and may have arisen after the last colonoscopy.

Impress your attending

How often would you repeat a colonoscopy after finding a hyperplastic polyp?

Hyperplastic polyps, as seen in this patient, are often in the rectosigmoid area and are usually less than 5mm. They are felt to confer no additional risk of colon cancer, and a 10-year screening interval is therefore adequate.

Which adenomas have the highest malignant potential?

Adenomas with 'advanced' features (i.e., more villous than tubular component) are felt to have higher malignant potential. Therefore, villous adenomas have the greatest malignant potential and tubular adenomas the least; tubulovillous adenomas are intermediate.

Case 4

A 56-year-old woman was admitted for a community-acquired pneumonia. An initial chest radiograph showed a consolidation in the right lower lobe. The patient could not tolerate oral medications secondary to nausea and vomiting, and therefore was subsequently admitted. The patient's presenting symptoms of cough, chest pain with deep inspiration, and fever had improved by hospital day 2. By day 3, the patient was tolerating a diet and was discharged home on a course of levofloxacin 750mg for an additional 4 days, with a plan for a repeat chest radiograph in 6 weeks.

Three days later, the patient returns to the hospital with abdominal pain. Her pain is located in the lower abdomen and began 1 day prior. She describes it as crampy in nature, with no radiation and no specific aggravating or relieving factors. She gives the pain a rating of 7/10 at worst, and says the only other associated symptom is diarrhea. She has had about 10 watery bowel movements since yesterday – symptoms she has never had before. She has not eaten in the past 24 hours.

What is your differential diagnosis?

The differential diagnosis includes *Clostridium difficile* colitis, other infectious colitis, gastroenteritis, appendicitis, and medication side effect.

Physical examination

Vitals Temperature 100.5°F, HR 96 bpm, BP 105/64mmHg, oxygen saturation 99% on RA.

GEN Appears weak.

HEENT Dry mucous membranes. No scleral icterus. No lymphadenopathy.

CVS Normal S1, S2. No murmurs, rubs, or gallops.

RESP Bronchial breath sounds at the right lung base. Positive egophony at the right base.

ABD Diffuse tenderness throughout the abdomen. No rigidity, guarding, or rebound tenderness. Bowel sounds are slightly hyperactive. Rectal examination reveals an empty vault.

EXT Decreased skin turgor.

Does this narrow your differential diagnosis?

No. The physical examination findings can still point to any diagnosis.

What blood test(s) will you order?

CBC	**WBC**	15 x 10^3/μL
	Hemoglobin	15.1g/dL
	Hematocrit	39%
	Platelets	290 x 10^3μL

CHEM-6		
	Na	143mEq/L
	K	3.3mEq/L
	Cl	105mEq/L
	Bicarbonate	24mEq/L
	BUN	27mg/dL
	Creatinine	1.3mg/dL

In the setting of the patient's pneumonia, what does this WBC count mean?

The patient was recently discharged after starting an antibiotic course for pneumonia. It is important to check on her WBC trend during her previous hospital stay. The medical records reveal she was admitted with a WBC of 20 x 10^3/μL, and discharged when it was 11 x 10^3/μL. Now her WBC has come back up, this could suggest a new infectious process. Next you should look at the WBC differential, as a 'left shift' or increase in neutrophils can suggest an infectious etiology.

What other laboratory test will you order?

C. difficile toxin (enzyme immunoassay).

The test returns and is negative; however, this takes at least a few hours.

Imaging

Meanwhile, the emergency-room physician decides to proceed with imaging and obtains a CT scan of the abdomen and pelvis (Figures 8 and 9).

Describe what you see and read on

Figure 8 shows an axial view of the abdomen through the level of the iliac bones. Figure 9 is a coronal image at the level of the abdominal aorta. Oral contrast has been given and is only seen within the small bowel. Figure 9 demonstrates circumferential wall thickening of the ascending colon (red arrows). There is adjacent pericolonic fat stranding (Figure 8, yellow arrow). The descending colon appears normal without surrounding inflammation (white arrow). No fluid collections are seen. The visualized portions of the liver, spleen, and bladder are normal. The aorta is normal in caliber and course. The radiologist's diagnosis is colitis of the ascending colon.

The next step is to admit the patient and determine the cause of the colitis. The patient will be kept nil by mouth, placed on IV fluids, and empirically treated for *C. difficile colitis*. Stool culture, sensitivity, and fecal leukocytes are ordered along with follow-up laboratory tests in the morning. Later, you are called regarding the negative results of the *C. difficile* toxin assay.

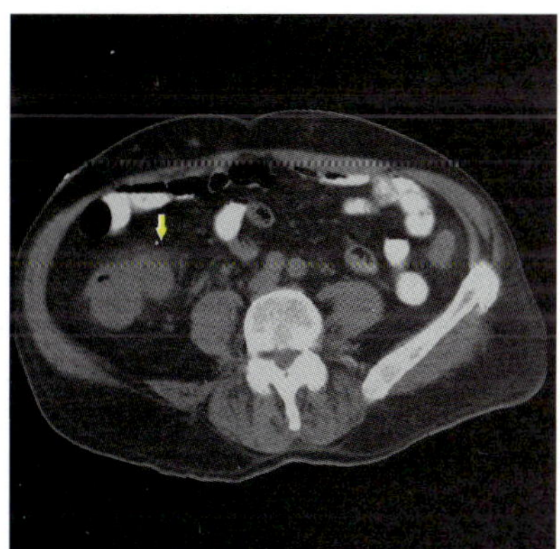

Figure 8.

What is the diagnosis, and how will you proceed?

Going through the differential diagnosis throughout this patient's stay brings out certain information. Despite keeping the

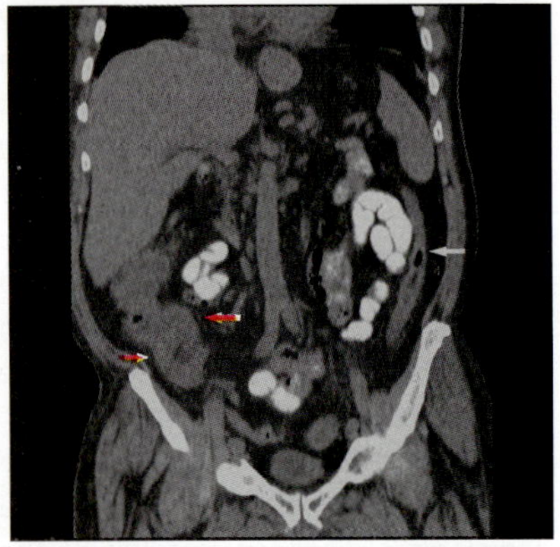

Figure 9.

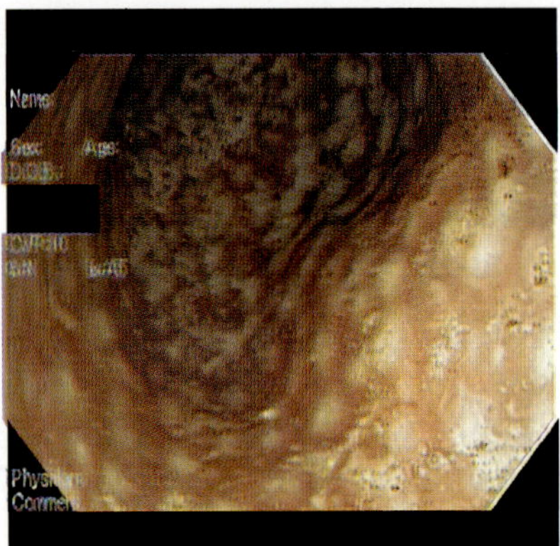

Figure 10.

This means osmotic causes are unlikely. A secretory diarrhea, as from a paraneoplastic syndrome, would not account for the leukocytosis or fever, and would be unlikely to generate such abdominal pain. A cholera toxin- or shiga toxin-producing organism could still be operant. Other food-borne gastroenteritides are also possible, except the patient's husband ate the exact same foods at home, and no one else she has been in contact with is ill.

C. difficile colitis secondary to antibiotic use is quite plausible, but the toxin assay was negative. Previous practice guidelines suggest the next step is to repeat the *C. difficile* toxin assay. However, new data suggest this will not increase the diagnostic yield [1]. You continue oral metronidazole 500mg three times a day, planning therapy for 10-14 days, and request flexible sigmoidoscopy or colonoscopy for further diagnostic evaluation. The colonoscopy findings are shown in Figure 10.

Describe what you see and read on

This endoscopic photo shows diffuse, superficial, yellowish plaques, commonly referred to as 'pseudomembranes.'

These findings are diagnostic of pseudomembranous colitis associated with *C. difficile*. The patient's risk factors include recent hospitalization and antibiotic therapy for pneumonia. No further diagnostic testing is needed. The patient should continue to improve with 10-14 days of oral metronidazole. She poses an infection risk for other family members, and should be counseled about proper hygiene, hand washing, and so on.

Clinical pearl

- Two enteric toxins are associated with *C. difficile:* toxin A and toxin B. The enzyme immunoassay commonly used to detect *C. difficile* toxin can detect both toxins. The test has specificity ranging from 92% to 99% but sensitivity is lower, ranging from 69% to 99% [2]. There can be a considerable false-negative rate. As a result, early endoscopy should be requested when the clinical suspicion is high but the initial toxin assay is negative. A stool *C. difficile* culture can also be obtained, but this takes considerable time. The diagnosis is more easily ruled in or out with prompt endoscopy. Stool

PCR testing is the most sensitive test, but is not clinically available at all centers.

Impress your attending

What are risk factors for Clostridium *difficile*- associated diarrhea?

Risk factors include recent antibiotic use, including fluoroquinolones, clindamycin, and broad-spectrum cephalosporins. Age older than 65 years, recent hospitalization, gastric acid suppression, and community-associated infection are other possible risk factors.

References

1. Deshpande A, Pasupuleti V, Patel P, *et al.* Repeat stool testing to diagnose *Clostridium difficile* infection using enzyme immunoassay does not increase diagnostic yield. *Clin Gastroenterol Hepatol* 2011; 9: 665-9.
2. Planche T, Aghaizu A, Holliman R, *et al.* Diagnosis of *Clostridium difficile* infection by toxin detection kits: a systematic review. *Lancet Infect Dis* 2008; 8: 777-84.

Case 5

A 36-year-old man presents to the local emergency department with abdominal pain. He describes the pain as crampy and intermittent, and it is periumbilical. Moving around makes the pain worse. More specifically, the area of maximum pain migrates as the patient rolls from side to side. Remaining immobile relieves the pain at times. At worst, he rates the pain as 7/10. The patient says he feels feverish at times.

Two days prior to these symptoms the patient saw his primary-care provider for excessive diarrhea, which was diagnosed as gastroenteritis. Those symptoms have improved but not abated. The patient feels his pain is different today, and has not been like this before. He has had a few episodes of vomiting without hematemesis. He has not traveled recently and none of his contacts are unwell. He says he had a sore throat a few days ago, and has felt lethargic since. He has previously been diagnosed with HIV but has not had recent blood work, and is not on HAART. He currently takes no medications.

What is your differential diagnosis?

The differential diagnosis includes gastroenteritis, mesenteric adenitis, colitis, viral syndrome, appendicitis, and neoplasm.

Physical examination

Vitals Temperature 99.5°F, HR 86 bpm, BP 125/75mmHg, oxygen saturation 98% on RA.

GEN Appears to be in mild distress.

HEENT Moist mucous membranes. No scleral icterus. No lymphadenopathy.

CVS Normal S1, S2. No murmurs, rubs, or gallops.

RESP Clear to auscultation.

ABD Abdomen is soft, but tender in the midline. No rigidity, guarding, or rebound tenderness. Bowel sounds are normal. Rotating the patient shifts the abdominal pain to the opposite direction.

EXT No clubbing, cyanosis, or edema.

Does this narrow your differential diagnosis?

Yes. The physical examination findings point more toward gastroenteritis, mesenteric adenitis, or perhaps a viral syndrome. The symptoms and physical examination findings do not fit colitis or appendicitis. Neoplasm is perhaps less likely as well.

What blood test(s) will you order?

CBC	**WBC**	$13 \times 10^3/\mu L$ with no left shift
	Hemoglobin	14.1g/dL

	Hematocrit	42%
	Platelets	$270 \times 10^3/\mu L$
CHEM-7		Normal
LFTs		Normal
CD4 count		$450mm^3$ (4 months prior)

Imaging

Meanwhile, the emergency-room physician proceeds with imaging in an attempt to narrow the differential diagnosis. He obtains a CT scan of the abdomen and pelvis (Figures 11 and 12).

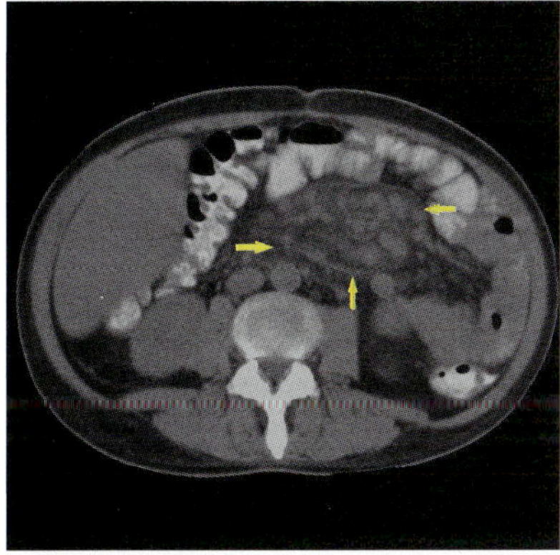

Figure 11.

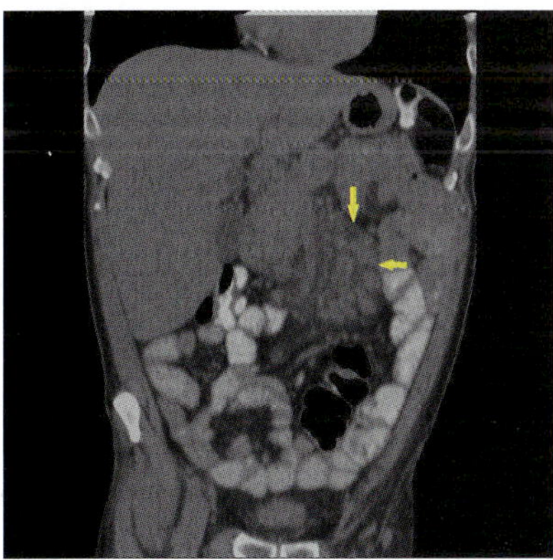

Figure 12.

Describe what you see and read on

Figure 11 shows an axial image of the abdomen through the inferior portion of the right lobe of the liver. Figure 12 shows a coronal image at the level of the pancreatic head and through the bulk of the liver. Oral contrast has been given and has opacified the bowel through the transverse colon. No IV contrast is present. Lymphadenopathy can be seen within the left upper quadrant with adjacent fat stranding (both images, yellow arrows). No fluid collection is seen. The lymph nodes measure up to 10mm in diameter. The visualized portions of the liver appear normal. The visualized small bowel and colon appear normal in size and course, without evidence of colitis or diverticulitis. The appendix is seen more inferiorly and is normal (not shown). There is no free fluid.

What is the diagnosis, and how will you proceed?

Going through the differential diagnosis and based on this patient's history, physical examination, and imaging findings, the adenopathy and stranding of the mesentery are concerning for mesenteric adenitis.

Management is based upon the patient's symptoms. First, the severity of his illness needs to be determined. As long as the patient does not show signs of volume depletion, significant electrolyte imbalance, or sepsis, then he can be managed as an outpatient with his primary-care physician. Antibiotics are often empirically started in moderately to severely ill patients. The most common organism involved with this diagnosis is *Yersinia enterocolitica*. Usual antibiotics include trimethopri sulfamethoxazole, third-generation cephalosporins, and fluoroquinolones.

You decide this patient is well enough to go home and does not need antibiotics. You arrange follow-up with the primary-care physician for next week. You advise the patient to take ibuprofen as needed and to keep hydrated.

Clinical pearls

- Although this patient presented with diffuse abdominal pain, patients with mesenteric adenitis typically exhibit right lower quadrant pain and can present with an upper respiratory tract infection just prior to these symptoms.
- Ingestion of raw pork can cause *Y. enterocolitica* infection and, therefore, travel and diet histories are important.

Impress your attending

In this patient with HIV infection, what underlying malignancy should you be concerned about?

Lymphoma remains in the differential diagnosis, but if the patient's symptoms resolve promptly with antibiotic and anti-inflammatory therapy, then repeat imaging is not needed. If his symptoms persist, the patient should have a follow-up CT scan to ensure the nodes regress.

Case 6

A 64-year-old woman with an 8-year history of gastroesophageal reflux presents to the emergency room with increasing chest pain over the past 3 weeks. She says the pain is in the epigastrium and radiates to the sternal region. She rates it at 5/10 at worst, and is pain-free a few hours following a meal or after taking over-the-counter antacids. She describes the pain as a dull burning pain and sometimes experiences a sour taste in her throat during the episodes. Occasionally she has a sensation of fullness in the substernal region with meals, which subsides with time. She has no dysphagia to solids or liquids. She has had no weight loss or change in appetite, but she does experience occasional postprandial nausea.

The patient presented to her primary-care physician 2 weeks previously. Her physician ordered an outpatient cardiac work-up, on which the patient demonstrated a normal electrocardiogram and stress test. The patient has a pacemaker because of symptomatic bradycardia in the past. Her cholesterol panel showed her low-density lipoprotein cholesterol level to be at goal for her risk factors.

The patient has no other associated symptoms and lives an active lifestyle, playing tennis regularly. She goes to the gym to lift weights and keep fit. She is currently taking a proton-pump inhibitor.

What is your differential diagnosis?

The differential diagnosis includes gastroesophageal reflux, esophageal stricture, hiatal hernia, and cardiac chest pain.

Physical examination

Vitals Temperature 97.8°F, HR 76 bpm, BP 140/80mmHg, oxygen saturation 99% on RA.

GEN The patient looks well, and appears of normal stature and build.

HEENT Moist mucous membranes. No scleral icterus. No lymphadenopathy.

CVS Normal S1, S2. No murmurs, rubs, or gallops.

RESP Clear to auscultation.

ABD No abdominal protrusion. Abdomen is soft and non-tender. No rigidity, guarding, or rebound tenderness. Bowel sounds are normal.

EXT No clubbing, cyanosis, or edema.

MSK Palpation over the chest wall does not reproduce the pain. Normal-appearing muscle bulk.

Does this narrow your differential diagnosis?

No. The physical examination findings have not helped to narrow the differential diagnosis significantly.

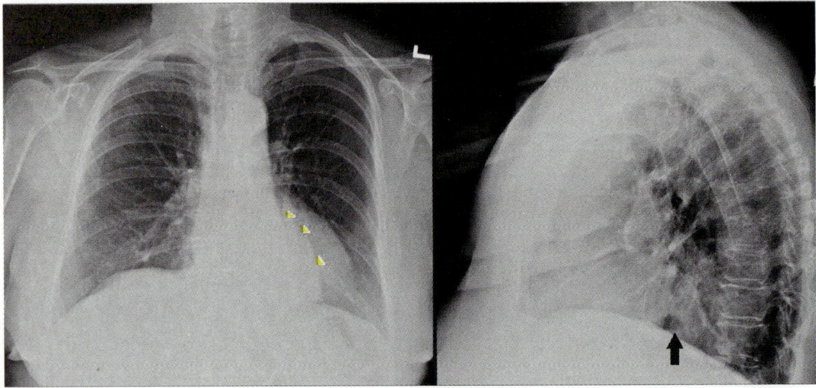

Figure 13.

What is the next step?

Although the symptoms are less likely to be cardiac, precautionary measures must still be taken not to miss a cardiac diagnosis. The next step is to obtain an EKG, blood work, and imaging. The EKG returns as normal.

What blood test(s) will you order?

CBC	WBC	8.5 x 10^3/μL
	Hemoglobin	14.4g/dL
	Hematocrit	41%
	Platelets	250 x 10^3/μL
CHEM-7		Normal
Troponin		Not elevated
CK-MB		Normal

What imaging test will you order?

A chest radiograph (Figure 13) is obtained to rule out obvious causes of the pain.

Describe what you see and read on

The posteroanterior view (left) shows the trachea to be central. The cardiac silhouette is normal in size. The lung parenchyma is clear. There is no venous congestion, pleural fluid, or pneumothorax. There is a retrocardiac opacity (yellow arrowheads) with, on the lateral view (right), an air-fluid level (black arrow). Findings are consistent with a hiatal hernia of at least 8cm in its greatest dimension.

The patient has a working diagnosis of a large hiatal hernia. Given she has a longstanding history of reflux disease, further evaluation of the anatomy of the esophagus is indicated.

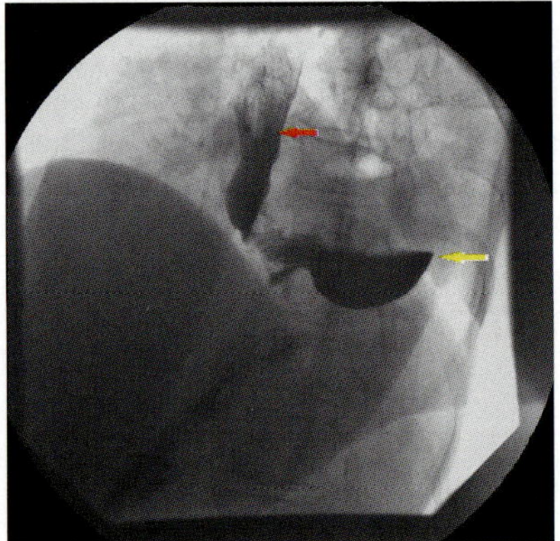

Figure 14.

Describe what you see and read on

This is an upper GI examination using liquid barium sulfate. The patient is in the steep right oblique position.

Barium is seen in the esophagus (red arrow) and stomach. Above the diaphragm, a wide-mouth hiatal hernia (yellow arrow) is seen projecting up to 5.5cm above the left hemidiaphragm.

The patient is kept on a clear liquid diet overnight. A GI consultation is obtained to rule out underlying neoplasia or dysplasia due to the longstanding reflux disease. An upper endoscopy is performed (Figure 15).

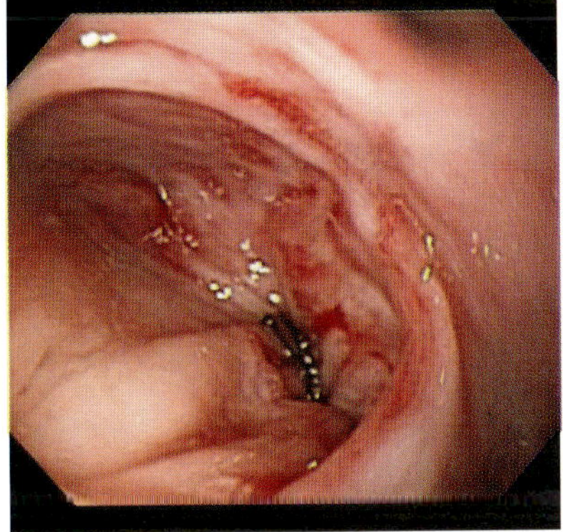

Figure 15.

Describe what you see and read on

The image shows a shallow Schatzki ring with esophagitis and/or trauma from retching (possibly during endoscopy). Gastric folds are present in the chest above the diaphragmatic 'pinch.' The 5cm hernia sack seen on X-ray begins at the bottom left of the photo and extends out of view to the left.

How will you proceed?

Making the diagnosis was straightforward. In fact, it was made on the initial chest radiograph. Most patients are asymptomatic, and a work-up for this diagnosis is done as an outpatient. However, our patient was experiencing worsening symptoms while on proton-pump inhibitors. The patient had a couple of risk factors for the development of a hernia, including the repetitive strain of working out at the gym and longstanding acid reflux. Treatment can be either medical or surgical.

It should be noted that the patient had considerable pain — more than would be expected from reflux alone. Indeed, she required hospitalization because of poorly controlled pain. In this setting, gastric torsion or volvulus should be considered, and inpatient surgical consultation is reasonable. This diagnosis cannot always be made with endoscopy. If the endoscopy and upper GI series are equivocal, CT scanning can be helpful.

The patient responded promptly to increased acid-suppression therapy. She was discharged on medical therapy with an outpatient follow-up appointment with a surgeon to discuss her options.

Clinical pearls

- Most hiatal hernias are asymptomatic, but a large fraction are associated with symptomatic reflux.
- Medical treatment usually entails proton-pump inhibitors.
- Surgical management usually involves reducing the herniated stomach below the diaphragm, repairing the crural defect, and fundoplication to help prevent future reflux.

Impress your attending

What are the different types of hiatal hernias?

- Type 1: sliding hiatal hernia — occurs when the stomach slides in and out of the hiatus.
- Type 2: paraesophageal hernia — occurs when part of the stomach squeezes through the hiatus and lies next to the esophagus.
- Type 3: combined sliding and paraesophageal hernia.
- Type 4: complex paraesophageal hernia — an esophageal hernia with other abdominal contents.

Case 7

A 42-year-old man presents to the local emergency department with a 2-day history of abdominal pain. The pain is located in the epigastric region. The patient describes it as being constant and burning in nature, and radiating in a band-like fashion to his back. He grades the pain as 7/10 in severity. Moving his torso and eating aggravate the pain, while lying still relieves it. The patient denies nausea, vomiting, or diarrhea. He does not take any medications, except for a multivitamin tablet. He says he has never had this pain before.

Socially, the patient drinks a couple of beers every night. He had a little more than usual the other night, but has not had anything to drink for the past couple of days because of stock issues at the local liquor store. Generally, he does not have abdominal pain after meals.

What is your differential diagnosis?

The differential diagnosis includes acute pancreatitis, cholelithiasis, and peptic ulcer disease.

Physical examination

Vitals Temperature 101.5°F, HR 112 bpm, BP 115/68mmHg, oxygen saturation 98% on RA.

GEN Unkempt appearance.

HEENT Dry mucous membranes. Scleral icterus. No lymphadenopathy.

CVS Normal S1, S2. No murmurs, rubs, or gallops.

RESP Clear to auscultation.

ABD Diffuse tenderness in the epigastric region.

The patient has voluntary guarding. Bowel sounds are hypoactive. There is good rectal tone and only trace stool in the vault, which is guaiac-negative.

EXT Decreased skin turgor.

Skin No erythema noted in the flanks or periumbilical region.

Does this narrow your differential diagnosis?

Yes. The history and physical examination indicate a classic presentation of acute, alcohol-induced pancreatitis.

What blood test(s) will you order?

CBC	WBC	13 x 10^3/μL
	Hemoglobin	15.1g/dL
	Hematocrit	39.4%
	Platelets	300x10^3/μL
CHEM-6	Na	142mEq/L
	K	3.5mEq/L
	Cl	104mEq/L
	Bicarbonate	24mEq/L
	BUN	23mg/dL
	Creatinine	1.1mg/dL
LFTs	AST	70 units/L
	ALT	46 units/L

Alkaline phosphatase	90 units/L
Total bilirubin	2.2mg/dL
Lipase	570 units/L

The patient is presenting with a clinical picture of pancreatitis. What is the next step in determining the etiology?

The laboratory data help build the case that this is pancreatitis. The patient is presenting with jaundice and elevated LFTs. The two most common causes of pancreatitis in the Western world are gallstones and alcohol. Alcohol-induced pancreatitis is seen somewhat more often in men than women, but gallstone pancreatitis is still more common. The higher AST than ALT level suggests recent alcohol use, and the relatively low lipase level (given the degree of the patient's symptoms) also suggests alcoholic pancreatitis. Imaging is not always needed in pancreatitis, but is frequently used to assess for etiologies and complications. The patient's LFTs indicate mild transaminitis and elevated alkaline phosphatase, which could suggest an obstructed biliary tree. As a result, you order a right upper quadrant ultrasound (Figure 16).

Describe what you see and read on

A limited sagittal view of the right upper quadrant shows a non-distended gallbladder without gallstones (white arrow). The gallbladder wall is not thickened. There is no pericholecystic fluid. The common bile duct measures 4mm (not shown) and is without stones. However, the common duct tapers abruptly

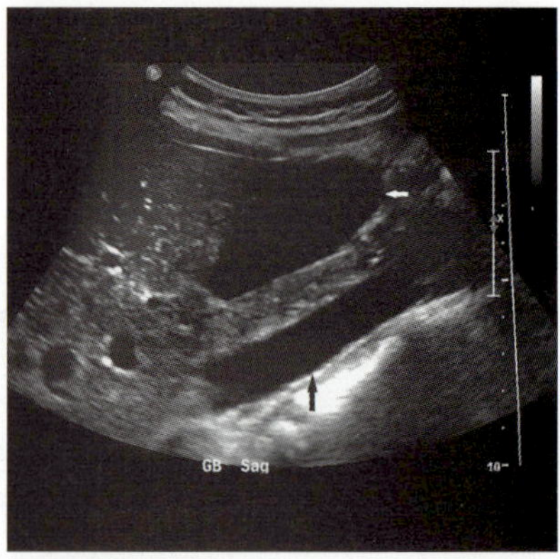

Figure 16.

The ultrasound did not help determine the etiology for this patient's pancreatitis, but has made you think there is some process occurring in the head of the pancreas causing obstruction of both the common bile and pancreatic ducts. Regardless, the patient is admitted for further care and work-up.

How will you initially manage this patient?

First, you must decide how unwell the patient is. Based on the laboratory data and examination, he seems to have a mild episode of pancreatitis. He should be taken care of on the regular medical ward. Initial management will include not feeding the patient, placing him on IV fluids, and pain control as needed.

You can start with 150-200mL/h of normal saline, and use 2-4mg of morphine every 4-6 hours as needed. Although morphine can increase pressure within the sphincter of Oddi, thus potentially worsening biliary outflow, narcotics are necessary for pain control and have not been shown to affect the course of acute pancreatitis.

The next morning the patient appears better, but given your concern about the abrupt narrowing of the common bile duct, you decide to order a CT scan of the abdomen for further assessment of the pancreas (Figures 17 and 18). This was conducted with oral contrast only. The image shows the following.

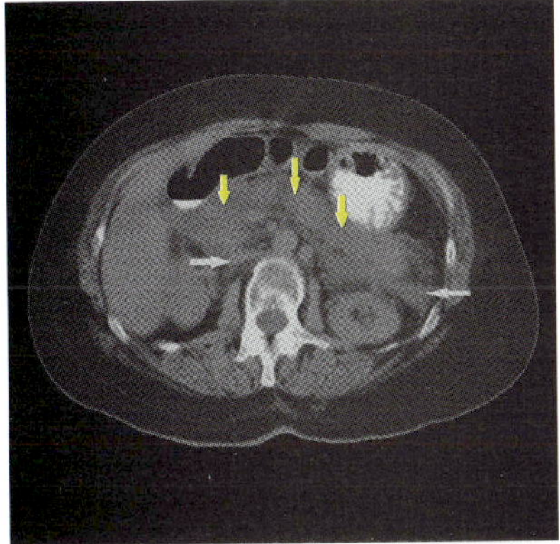

Figure 17.

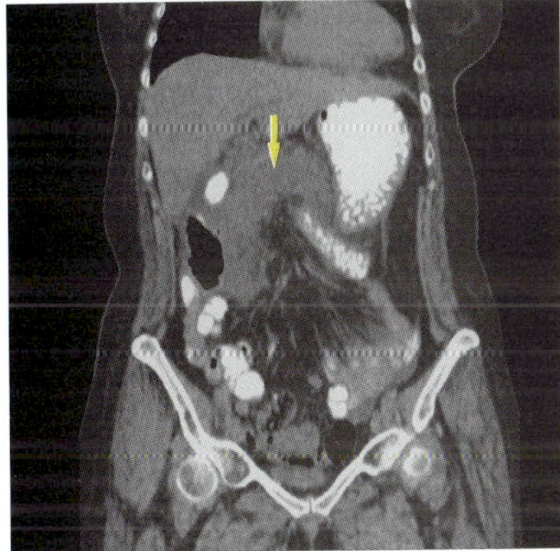

Figure 18.

Describe what you see and read on

The CT axial image at the level of the pancreas (Figure 17) demonstrates an edematous pancreas throughout its entire course of the head, neck, body, and tail (yellow arrows). Peripancreatic fat stranding is identified (white arrows). No cysts are seen. The coronal image (Figure 18) demonstrates an edematous head of the pancreas (arrow). The common bile duct is not visualized on this image. No masses are identified and there is no visible adenopathy. The surrounding loops of bowel appear normal in size and caliber. Minimal free fluid is noted inferior to the pancreas on the coronal images. There is no soft-tissue anasarca.

What is the next step?

No mass was seen, and you later confirm with the patient that he has no constitutional symptoms (weight loss or fatigue) to suggest malignancy. The patient says he is feeling better and his vital signs are within normal limits. Even so, you need to check how often the patient has been requesting pain medication, as that can mask symptoms. You see he only requested morphine once overnight. You also notice in his laboratory data that his lipase has decreased by 50%. The patient allows you to examine his abdomen fully and you notice decreased tenderness on examination.

A few hours later, the patient feels hungry and asks for food, which is a good sign for improvement. The patient should be started on a clear liquid diet later that day or perhaps the next, and advanced as tolerated. Once the patient is tolerating a diet orally and is off IV pain medication, he can be safely discharged home.

What caused this patient's pancreatitis?

This patient's symptoms were caused by binge drinking, which brought on acute, alcohol-induced pancreatitis, mostly involving the head of the pancreas. The head has become edematous and is compressing the biliary system. You recommend the patient does not drink as much in the future.

If you keep this patient in hospital any longer, what is he at risk of?

Being a regular drinker, the patient is at risk from alcohol withdrawal. Although symptoms of this condition were not elicited from the history, all physicians must be aware of this complication. Alcohol withdrawal can prolong a hospital stay by days, and is associated with significant morbidity and mortality.

Clinical pearl

- Causes of pancreatitis ("I GET SMASHED"):
  - **I**diopathic;
  - **G**allstones;
  - **E**thanol;
  - **T**rauma;
  - **S**teroids;
  - **M**umps;
  - **A**utoimmune (also includes polyarteritis nodosa and lupus);
  - **S**corpion sting;
  - **H**ypercalcemia, **H**yperlipidemia (triglycerides usually >1,000mg/dL), **H**ypothermia;
  - **E**RCP;
  - **D**rugs.

Impress your attending

What are the Ranson criteria?

This is a scoring method to stratify the risk of mortality and severity of pancreatitis.

Table 1. Ranson criteria.

On admission	48 h after admission
Age >55 years	Serum calcium <8mg/dL
WBC >16 x 10^3/μL	Hematocrit fall >10%
Blood glucose >200mg/dL	Hypoxemia PO_2 <60mmHg
Serum AST >250 units/L	BUN >5mg/dL after IV fluids
Serum LDH >350 units/L	Base deficit >4mEq/L
	Sequestration of fluids >6L

Each of the above parameters in Table 1 is worth 1 point. A total score of 3 or higher means severe pancreatitis is likely. A score of less than 3 means severe pancreatitis is unlikely:

- Score 0-2: 2% mortality.
- Score 3 or 4: 15% mortality.
- Score 5 or 6: 40% mortality.
- Score 7 or 8: 100% mortality.

Case 8

A 74-year-old man presents to the emergency room with upper abdominal and chest pain, along with shortness of breath. For the past 2-3 days the patient has had general malaise, weakness, and loss of appetite. He has vomited at least eight times in the past 24 hours, and says that after the last episode of vomiting he developed intense upper abdominal and retrosternal pain. He describes it as being sharp, 10/10 in severity, and is only now starting to ease. There is no radiation. As the pain is new, he cannot say what aggravates or relieves it. There are no other associated symptoms such as hematemesis. He has had normal bowel movements and his stools are brown. His past medical history is significant for peripheral vascular disease and high cholesterol. The patient drinks occasionally, is a former smoker, and has no history of gastric ulcers.

What is your differential diagnosis?

The differential diagnosis includes gastroenteritis, pyloric channel ulcer, perforated esophagus, aortic dissection, and viral syndrome.

Physical examination

Vitals	Temperature 100.5°F, HR 110 bpm, BP 100/60mmHg, respiratory rate 26 breaths per minute, oxygen saturation 91% on RA.
GEN	Appears in agony.
HEENT	Moist mucous membranes. No scleral icterus. No lymphadenopathy.
CVS	Tachycardic. Normal S1, S2. No murmurs, rubs, or gallops.
RESP	Dullness to percussion at both bases. Decreased breath sounds on the right. Decreased vocal resonance on the right.
ABD	Abdomen is tender in the epigastric region. No rigidity, guarding, or rebound tenderness. Bowel sounds are normal.
EXT	No edema.
MSK	Palpation over the sternum reveals crepitus.

Does this narrow your differential diagnosis?

Yes. The physical examination findings point more toward a pneumothorax. Given the history of vomiting with subsequent severe pain, an esophageal perforation or rupture is likely.

You order blood work while the radiology department mobilizes technicians to obtain a portable chest X-ray

CBC	WBC	18.5 x 10^3/μL with a left shift
	Hemoglobin	14.3g/dL
	Hematocrit	41%
	Platelets	250x10^3/μL

CHEM-7	Na	142mEq/L
	K	3.1mEq/L
	Cl	105mEq/L
	Bicarbonate	23mEq/L
	BUN	30mg/dL
	Creatinine	1.4mg/dL
	Glucose	92mg/dL
Troponin		Not elevated

This blood work is concerning, indicating an infectious process. The next step is to obtain blood cultures right away.

A chest radiograph is obtained (Figure 19).

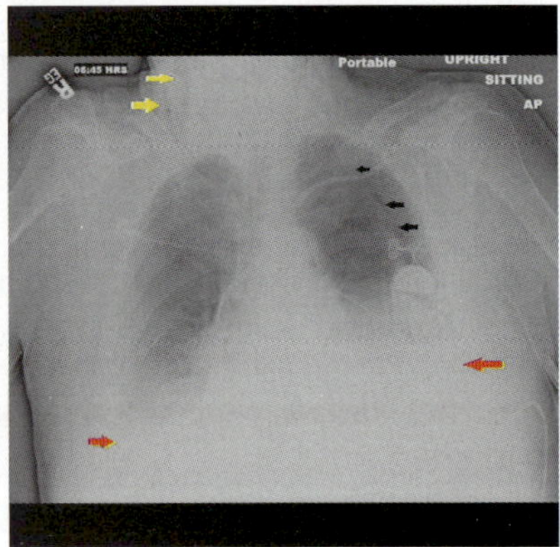

Figure 19.

Describe what you see and read on

A portable upright radiograph is obtained. The trachea is slightly to the right of the midline. The cardiac silhouette is large. A dual-lead pacemaker is present over the left hemithorax with wires extending to overlie the heart. A moderate left-sided pneumothorax is noted without tension (black arrows). There is gas in the soft tissues of the neck bilaterally (yellow arrows). Increased attenuation is present at the lung bases, left greater than right, consistent with bilateral pleural effusions (red arrows).

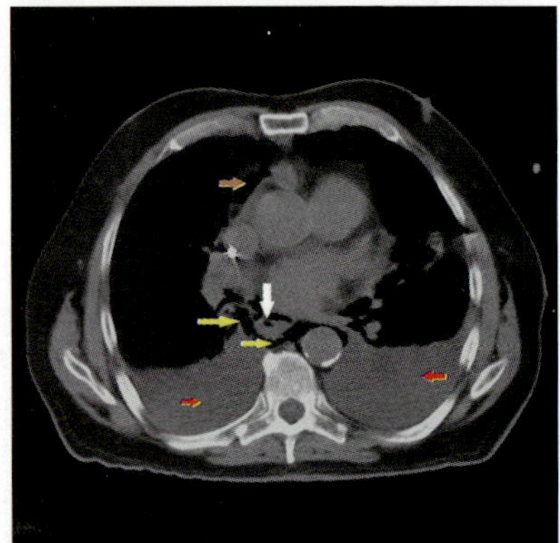

Figure 20.

Given the large pneumothorax, the next step is to call for a surgical consultation to place chest tubes. The surgeons order a CT scan of the chest to allow better assessment (Figure 20).

Describe what you see and read on

A single axial image at the level of the origin of the ascending aorta is shown. There are bilateral moderate-sized pleural effusions (red arrows). In the posterior mediastinum, locules/tracks of low attenuation (which measure air density) are present (yellow arrows). These tracks of air seem to be more centered along the posterior aspect of the esophagus (white arrow). The air then tracks anterolaterally to the heart (brown arrow). Sequential images show the air tracks superiorly into the neck (not shown).

Given the findings of pneumomediastinum and a major focus of air arising posterior to the distal esophagus, the next step is to rule out an esophageal perforation. The examination of choice is an esophagram using fluoroscopy. Because of the urgency of this study and the implications of the diagnosis, you physically wheel the patient to the fluoroscopy suite. You then find a radiologist to perform the study. The patient is positioned and the study is started (Figure 21).

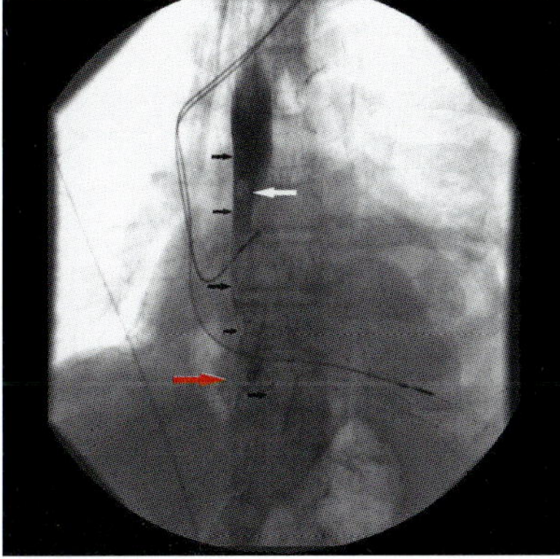

Figure 21.

Describe what you see and read on

The patient is examined in the supine position and given multiple sips of contrast through a straw. The proximal esophagus is distended with contrast. An air bubble is present in the mid-esophagus (white arrow). At the distal third of the esophagus, inferior to the level of the pacemaker lead heading to the right ventricle, contrast is heading in a lateral direction to the right (red arrow). The patient is slightly rotated to the left to place him in an oblique view to demonstrate that contrast is heading in a posterior direction (not shown). The black arrows mark the esophageal wall.

This examination would ideally be done in the upright, lateral, and oblique views. This patient is very ill and therefore proper technique could not be utilized.

What is the next step?

You have now confirmed this patient has an esophageal perforation along with a large pneumothorax, and bilateral pleural effusions. He has an elevated WBC, low BP, and rising temperature. He most likely has a polymicrobial infection within the effusions from esophageal and gastric contents.

At this point, the next step would be to take the patient to the operating room to repair the esophageal perforation. The usual approach includes a primary repair, with or without reinforcement, mediastinal debridement, and possible pleural drainage if an effusion is present. The patient will be monitored postoperatively in the intensive care unit with serial chest radiographs to monitor his pneumothorax, effusions, and pneumomediastinum. He should also be placed on broad-spectrum antibiotics. His vital

signs and mental status will need to be monitored carefully.

Clinical pearls

- The final diagnosis for this patient's esophageal perforation is Boerhaave's syndrome. This was caused by a sudden increase in intraesophageal pressure combined with negative intrathoracic pressure from vomiting.
- Other causes of esophageal perforation include ingestion of foreign bodies and medical instrumentation, such as after endoscopy or transesophageal echocardiography.
- Cervical esophageal repairs can sometimes be managed conservatively. Thoracic esophageal ruptures require urgent surgery, and any delay increases the chance of mortality.
- Endoscopy has no role in the diagnosis of spontaneous

esophageal perforations. The air insufflated during endoscopy can make symptoms worse.

Impress your attending

What type of contrast would you use in the fluoroscopy study for this patient?

In general, two types of contrast are used: barium-based and water-soluble. Initially, a water-soluble contrast would be used in a patient with suspected esophageal rupture. Barium is essentially toxic outside of the aerodigestive tract. Water-soluble contrast is somewhat irritating, but does not cause a significant reaction. If the study is negative with a water-soluble contrast, barium can be used for further evaluation; the sensitivity of detecting a perforation increases because of barium's greater density.

Case 9

A 24-year-old man presents to the emergency room complaining of abdominal pain. He says the pain started in the region of the umbilicus, but has slowly migrated and is now more localized in the right lower abdomen. He describes it as a vague constant pain over the general region. He rates the pain as 6/10 in severity, although it worsens to 10/10 when he coughs or performs other movements. Staying still keeps the pain at bay. He has lost his appetite and today developed nausea and vomiting. He has never had this pain before. His bowel movements have become irregular. His friend says the patient has been feverish and lethargic. None of his contacts are unwell and he has not eaten anything that may have been spoiled.

What is your differential diagnosis?

The differential diagnosis includes appendicitis, ileitis, cecal diverticulitis, and colitis.

Physical examination

Vitals Temperature 100.8°F, HR 86 bpm, BP 130/85mmHg, respiratory rate 20, oxygen saturation 98% on RA.

GEN The patient looks ill.

HEENT Dry mucous membranes. No scleral icterus. No lymphadenopathy.

CVS Normal S1, S2. No murmurs, rubs, or gallops.

RESP Clear to auscultation.

ABD The abdomen is tender 2-3 inches in the superomedial direction from the anterior superior iliac spine toward the umbilicus. No rigidity or guarding. Bowel sounds are normal.

EXT No clubbing or edema.

Does this narrow your differential diagnosis?

Yes. The history and physical examination are classic for a diagnosis of appendicitis. Ileitis can still be in the differential diagnosis. Cecal diverticulitis is less likely, as cecal diverticula are uncommon and diverticulitis is quite rare in this age group. Colitis is still in the differential diagnosis, but the history favors appendicitis.

What blood test(s) will you order?

CBC	WBC	14.5 x 10^3/μL
	Hemoglobin	14.6g/dL
	Hematocrit	42%
	Platelets	275 x 10^3/μL
CHEM-7	Na	140mEq/L
	K	3.6mEq/L
	Cl	102mEq/L
	Bicarbonate	24mEq/L
	BUN	20mg/dL
	Creatinine	1.3mg/dL
	Glucose	95mg/dL

What imaging test will you order?

With patients lining up to get a CT scan, you opt to begin with a radiograph of the abdomen. Under indications you click the first option under clinical symptoms, "abdominal distension." The image obtained is shown in Figure 22.

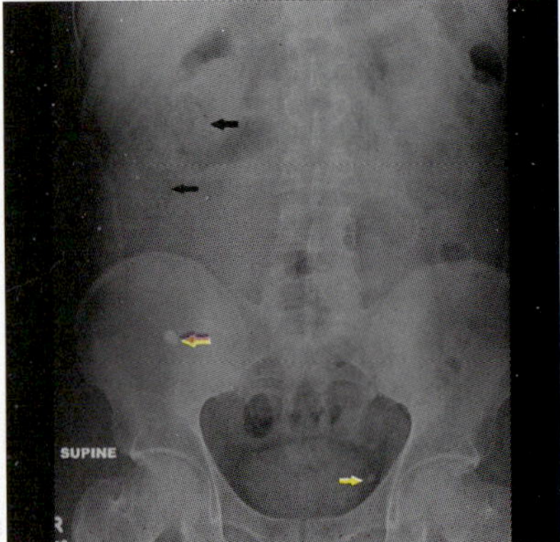

Figure 22.

Describe what you see and read on

This supine view of the abdomen shows a moderate volume of fecal material (black arrows) in the vicinity of the hepatic flexure of the colon and transverse colon. There are no abnormally dilated loops of bowel. There is no evidence of pneumoperitoneum. There are no masses or visceromegaly. Left-sided pelvic phleboliths are noted (yellow arrow). There is an oval calcification projecting over the right lower quadrant and the right iliac bone, measuring 1.3 x 0.9cm (brown arrow). This could be a calcified lymph node or an appendicolith. (Additional views demonstrated this did not significantly change in position with respect to the bone, suggesting a bone island is more likely.)

Your patient says the pain is getting worse and asks for more pain medication. After re-examining the patient, you feel that his abdomen is more tender. You proceed with a CT scan (Figures 23 and 24).

Describe what you see and read on

Axial (Figure 23) and coronal (Figure 24) images of the abdomen and pelvis are shown through the appendix. Both oral and IV contrast are administered. In the right lower quadrant, the appendix is distended (black arrow), fluid-filled, and contains a fecalith (red arrow).

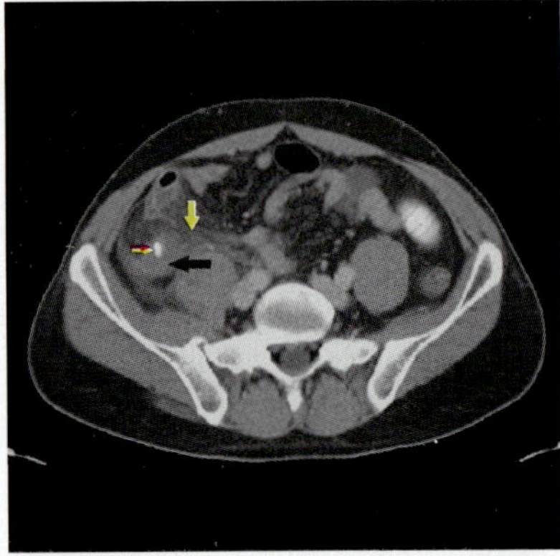

Figure 23.

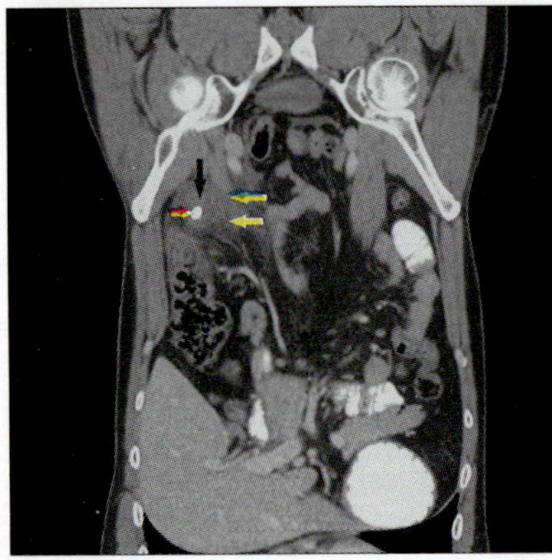

Figure 24.

There is a considerable degree of surrounding inflammatory reaction (yellow arrow) in the mesentery of the right lower quadrant. There is edema of the base of the cecum and terminal ileum, and of the right psoas muscle (green arrow). There is no focal abscess or extraluminal gas. The remainder of the visualized colon is unremarkable. Free fluid is noted within the pelvis and left paracolic gutter.

What is the next step?

A surgical consultation will need to be obtained, as this patient has clinical and radiographic findings consistent with acute appendicitis. He will need to be prepared for surgery. Adequate hydration, correction of electrolyte abnormalities, and preoperative antibiotics are key steps prior to surgery. This patient will need to go to the operating room as soon as possible to minimize the chance of progression to perforation.

In the operating room, the surgeon will proceed with either an open or laparoscopic appendectomy.

Clinical pearl

- Most patients with appendicitis present with a classic history. The reason for this is simple physiology. The visceral organs are not innervated with somatic pain fibers. As the inflammation progresses, the involvement of the overlying parietal peritoneum near the appendix causes localized tenderness in the right lower quadrant. This is reflected during abdominal, rectal, and pelvic examinations.

Impress your attending

What is the one important landmark and the three physical examination signs seen in various presentations of appendicitis?

- McBurney's point: a line drawn from the umbilicus to the anterior inferior iliac spine. The point is two-thirds of the way along the line and is where pain can eventually be localized.
- Rovsing's sign: palpation of the left lower quadrant causes pain in the right lower quadrant.
- Psoas sign: passive right hip extension causes pain in the right lower quadrant. This occurs when the inflamed appendix sits along the psoas muscle, which is indicative of a retrocecal appendix.
- Obturator sign: internal rotation and then flexion of the hip and knee elicits right lower quadrant pain. This indicates the appendix is in the pelvis.

Case 10

A 61-year-old woman arrives at the emergency department by ambulance. Emergency medical services were initially called for a "difficulty in breathing." When they arrived at the patient's home, she said she was being treated for a COPD exacerbation as an outpatient only. She could not stay in the hospital as she is her kids' only caretaker. Her symptoms have not improved over the past few days.

At her home the patient was initially bradycardic, but became somnolent and arrested while en route to the hospital, going into pulseless electrical activity. The patient was resuscitated with CPR and epinephrine for 2 minutes before regaining a pulse. By this point, the patient was intubated.

The emergency-room physician starts a work-up for respiratory failure. The patient has a 30-pack per year history of smoking. No other medical history is known. Laboratory tests and a chest radiograph are pending. IV fluids are started. The lactate comes back elevated at 7.8mmol/L. At this point, the emergency-room physician orders a surgical/GI consultation. Your attending asks you to see the patient as a consult.

As you walk to the emergency room, what is your differential diagnosis?

Given this patient's history, the elevated lactate level is probably a result of hypoperfusion secondary to shock and cardiopulmonary arrest. Ischemia and bowel infarction are other possibilities. Other causes of lactic acidosis (but not pertinent to this patient) include metformin use, alcoholism, HIV, and malignancy such as lymphoma.

The patient is unable to provide you with additional information as she is sedated and intubated. There are no family members at the bedside. There is no additional information in the electronic medical record, apart from her recent discharge for a COPD exacerbation.

Physical examination

Vitals Afebrile, HR 104 bpm, BP 100/55mmHg, oxygen

saturation 99% on mechanical ventilation.

GEN Currently sedated. Ill-appearing.

HEENT No scleral icterus.

CVS Normal S1, S2. No murmurs, rubs, or gallops.

RESP Faint expiratory wheeze, but otherwise clear to auscultation.

ABD Soft and non-tender. No rigidity, guarding, or rebound tenderness. Bowel sounds are hyperactive. Rectal examination reveals an empty

	vault with no blood on the glove.	
EXT	No edema.	

Blood test results

CBC	WBC	$12.7 \times 10^3/\mu L$
	Hemoglobin	10.7g/dL
	Hematocrit	34.8%
	Platelets	$207 \times 10^3/\mu L$
CHEM-7	Na	143mEq/L
	K	4.7mEq/L
	Cl	107mEq/L
	Bicarbonate	19mEq/L
	BUN	52mg/dL
	Creatinine	1.2mg/dL
	Glucose	99mg/dL
LFTs	AST	639 units/L
	ALT	985 units/L
	Alkaline phosphatase	60 units/L
	Total bilirubin	0.5mg/dL
Lactate		7.8mmol/L
ABG	pH	7.24
	PaO_2	237mmHg
	(intubated on supplemental oxygen)	
	$PaCO_2$	36mmHg

What do these laboratory data suggest?

With the elevated lactate, low bicarbonate, and low pH on ABG, this patient has lactic acidosis. Given the elevated AST and ALT levels and normal alkaline phosphatase, these results point toward a hepatocellular process.

What imaging test will you order?

After examining the patient and reviewing the data, you need to rule out bowel infarction and mesenteric ischemia. Your test of choice is a CT angiogram of the abdomen and pelvis (Figures 25 and 26).

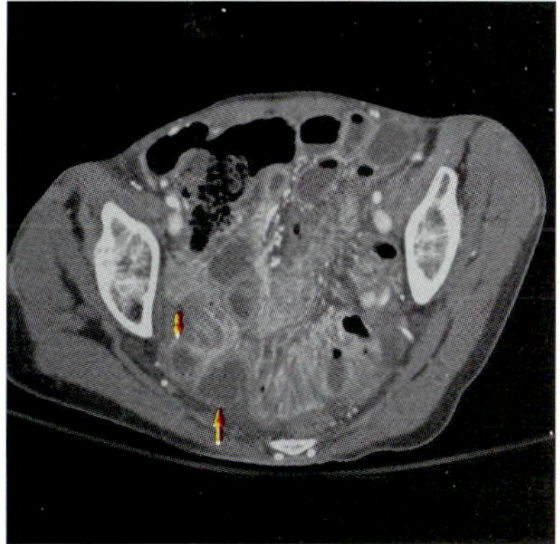

Figure 25.

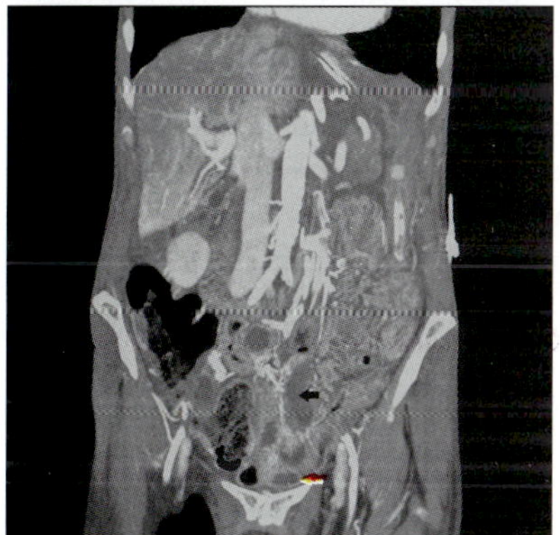

Figure 26.

Describe what you see and read on

Axial and coronal images with IV contrast are obtained. The visualized portions of the small bowel and colon are normal in size and course. There is diffuse enhancement of the small-bowel mucosa (Figure 25, red arrows) and edema within the surrounding mesentery. Diffuse bowel wall thickening is seen (Figure 26, red arrow). There is accumulation of intraluminal fluid (black arrow). No pneumatosis or portal venous gas is identified. Free fluid is noted in the pelvis.

These findings are consistent with 'shock bowel' followed by aggressive fluid resuscitation. The liver enzyme abnormality is consistent with 'shock liver.'

From a GI standpoint, what is the next step in management?

The next step is supportive management. The bowel took an insult during the resuscitation and demonstrates marked edema from the reperfusion. The plan would be to continue with serial abdominal examinations, monitor lactate levels, and watch the patient for signs of infection. With regard to this patient's presenting respiratory difficulties, she should be treated as having acute respiratory failure secondary to a COPD exacerbation. She will require steroids, scheduled nebulizer treatments, and an antibiotic such as azithromycin.

Clinical pearls

- Shock bowel is a CT finding that suggests reversible mesenteric ischemia.
- Shock liver is a reversible cause of (often impressive) transaminase elevation in patients who have temporary hypoperfusion of the liver from arrhythmia, shock, or other sources of transient hypotension.

Impress your attending

What structures in the abdomen enhance in shocked bowel, and what structures decrease in attenuation?

- Enhanced: bowel wall, kidneys, mesentery, liver, and adrenal glands.
- Decreased: pancreas and spleen.

Case 11

A 54-year-old man presents to his primary-care physician's office complaining of weakness. He lives an active lifestyle and was previously healthy. He regularly visits the gym, where he used to run 2-3 miles without stopping. During the past few months, however, he has had to stop occasionally because he is fatigued sooner than usual. When asked to elaborate, he says he becomes short of breath and his legs feel ready to give out.

Apart from his exercise routine, he has not noticed changes in his other daily activities of living. His appetite is normal and his weight has been steady. He does not complain of abdominal pain or symptoms attributable to gastroesophageal reflux. He was screened for colon cancer at the age of 52 years and was noted to have nothing more than mild diverticular disease. His father was diagnosed with stage 3 colon cancer at the age of 56 years. The patient says his bowel movements are regular; he does not have bloody stools and his stool caliber is unchanged. Review of other pertinent symptoms reveals nothing to suggest a pulmonary or cardiac etiology.

Physical examination

Vitals Afebrile, HR 98 bpm, BP 135/70mmHg, oxygen saturation 95% on RA.

GEN Well-built, muscular man.

Hands Pale palmar creases. HEENT Pale conjunctivae.

CVS Normal S1, S2. No murmurs, rubs, or gallops.

RESP Clear to auscultation.

ABD Soft and non-tender. No rigidity, guarding, or rebound tenderness. Bowel sounds are normal. Rectal examination reveals brown stool (stool occult-positive). No visible hemorrhoids.

EXT No edema.

What diagnosis does the history and physical examination suggest?

The physical examination points toward anemia, and the heme-positive stool suggests a GI cause. The exertional dyspnea, pale conjunctivae and palmar creases are suggestive of this finding.

Given the patient feels alright overall and is functioning well at home, you advise him to not exercise until further test results are available. Being worried about his family history, you order a CT enterography as well.

What causes within the GI tract will cause an occult bleed?

The diagnosis suggests anemia with possible underlying malignancy.

What test(s) will you order?

CBC, TSH, fecal occult blood.

The patient has the blood work done 3 days later and the results arrive to you electronically. They show the following:

CBC	**WBC**	11 x 10^3/μL
	Hemoglobin	7.5g/dL
	Hematocrit	24.7%
	Platelets	450 x 10^3/μL
TSH		1.15mIU/L (normal range 0.3-3.0mIU/L)

Fecal occult blood	Two out of the three samples are positive

The patient also has a CT scan that day, for which the results are pending. After calling the patient to discuss the blood test results, you learn he is feeling slightly weaker. You advise him to be directly admitted to the hospital for a blood transfusion as a daytime procedure.

The CT results become available (Figures 27 and 28).

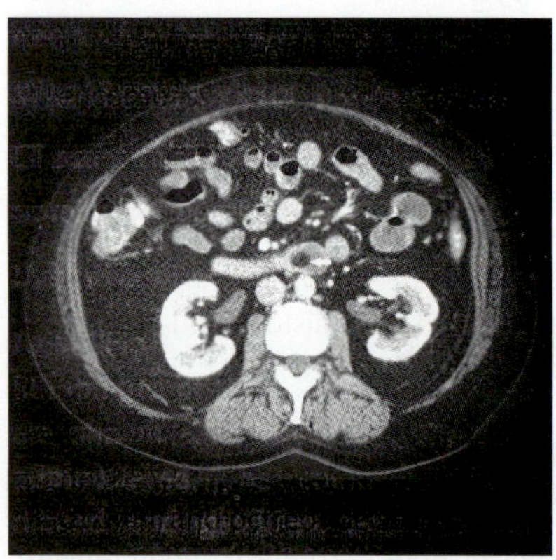

Figure 27.

Describe what you see and read on

The above scans demonstrate axial (Figure 27) and coronal (Figure 28) images of the abdomen and pelvis from this CT enterography with IV contrast. A tubular intraluminal filling defect measuring 4 x 1.5cm (white arrow) can be seen in the third portion of the duodenum.

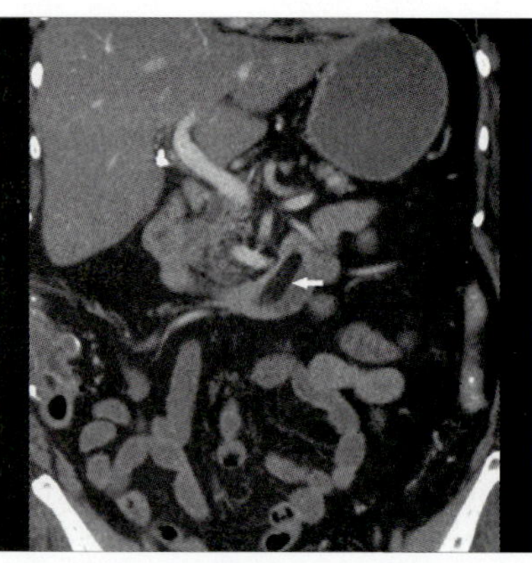

Figure 28.

The tubular structure appears to have the same density as fat. No other filling defects are seen in the bowel. The bowel itself is well distended with contrast and shows no wall thickening. The visualized colon is unremarkable with the exception of sigmoid diverticula (not shown). The stomach is normal. There is no adenopathy. The liver and kidneys are unremarkable.

Given these images and the patient's presenting history, what are you concerned about?

Without reading the entire radiology report, you are concerned about a duodenal tumor.

These results become available while the patient is at the day-stay suite receiving blood. The physician taking care of the patient calls for a GI consultation for "duodenal mass."

In the "Impression" of the radiology report, it states that this intraluminal mass is most likely a duodenal lipoma. However, given the degree of anemia, it would be wise to obtain an EGD for a biopsy. The patient is switched to being an "observation patient" (one most likely to be discharged in 24 hours) and kept nil by mouth overnight for an upper endoscopy the following morning.

The upper endoscopy results from a similar patient are shown in Figure 29.

Describe what you see and read on

A submucosal mass can be seen within the third portion of the duodenum. It is yellowish in color, and if pressed gently with biopsy forceps leaves a temporary indentation (the 'pillow sign'). This is characteristic of a submucosal lipoma.

Given the patient had severe anemia, probably as a result of the duodenal lipoma, endoscopic excision is planned for as an outpatient procedure. Removal by a snare during endoscopy is another option if subjectively the base of the lipoma is not broad. Otherwise, the risk of perforation is increased.

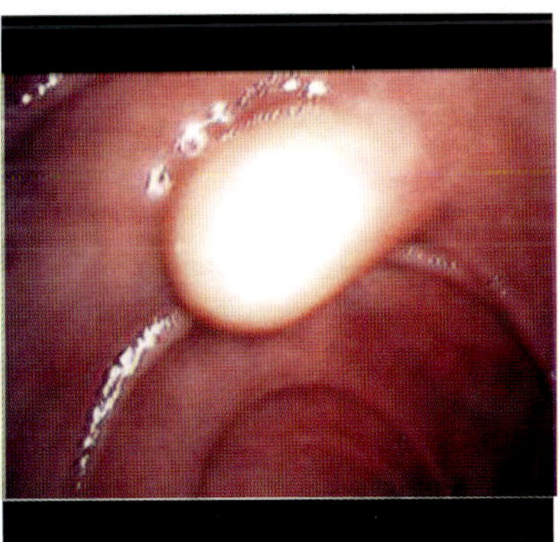

Figure 29.

Clinical pearls

- Duodenal lipomas are benign.
- In complicated cases of duodenal lipomas, signs and symptoms may include bleeding, pain, intussusception, obstruction, and obstructive jaundice.
- The mucosa overlying the lipoma is usually normal but can ulcerate, leading to bleeding and anemia in some cases.

Impress your attending

What are some other duodenal tumors?

- Adenocarcinoma, GI stromal tumors, and carcinoid tumors.
- Metastases - most commonly from breast or lung cancer, melanoma, or other GI malignancies.
- Lymphoma.

Case 12

A 65-year-old man presents to the clinic complaining of food getting stuck in his throat. His symptoms began about a year ago, at which time food became stuck only occasionally. At first he felt he just had a problem with liquids. Now, solid food is also getting stuck. He does not choke or feel unable to breathe when food is lodged. The patient became very concerned last weekend when he felt his BP medication was stuck in his throat.

Drinking water after a meal "makes the food go down my throat," he says. He has experienced no weight loss or change in appetite. His main concern is he has to keep drinking water to keep his throat clear. "Is it all in my head?" asks the patient. "My wife says I have bad breath more often than not." The patient also says he was admitted to the hospital with pneumonia 6 months ago

What is your differential diagnosis?

The differential diagnosis includes head/neck cancer, Zenker's diverticulum, traction diverticula, and globus.

Physical examination

Vitals Afebrile, HR 68 bpm, BP 155/84mmHg, oxygen saturation 98% on RA.

GEN No obvious distress. Hands No clubbing or muscle wasting.

H+N No scleral icterus. No adenopathy. No asymmetry within the oropharynx. Trachea is in the midline. Visual inspection of swallowing a glass of water looks normal and does not reproduce symptoms.

CVS Normal S1, S2. No murmurs, rubs, or gallops.

RESP Clear to auscultation.

ABD Soft and non-tender. No rigidity, guarding, or rebound tenderness. Bowel sounds are present. Rectal examination reveals brown stool.

EXT No edema.

What blood test(s) will you order?

No blood tests are needed.

What imaging test will you order?

Barium swallow or esophagram. These tests are the same but have different names.

What would you advise the patient regarding the test in terms of preparation?

Ideally the patient should eat nothing for a few hours prior to the examination. However, given the differential diagnosis, it would be ideal to have him eat nothing overnight to potentially keep his throat clear.

On the day of the examination, the patient will drink liquid barium, swallow a barium pill, and swallow barium-coated solids (often marshmallows or bread).

The images obtained are shown in Figure 30.

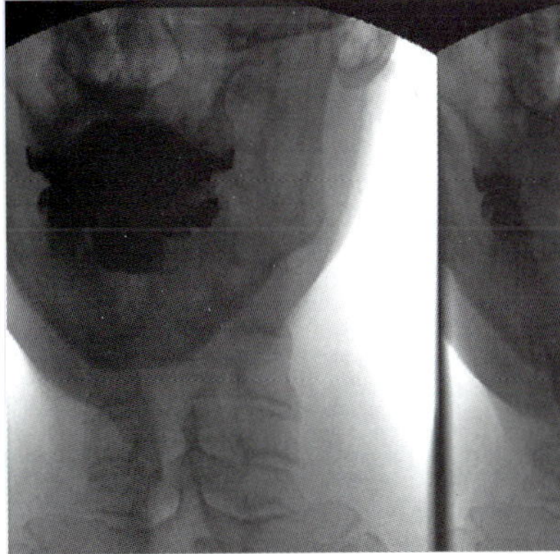

Figure 30.

Describe what you see and read on

These images show anteroposterior views of the upper chest and neck. The scout view (left) does not demonstrate abnormal osseous lesions. Barium contrast is present in the patient's mouth. The initial swallow (right) demonstrates a well-distended cervical esophagus. Further images are shown in Figure 31.

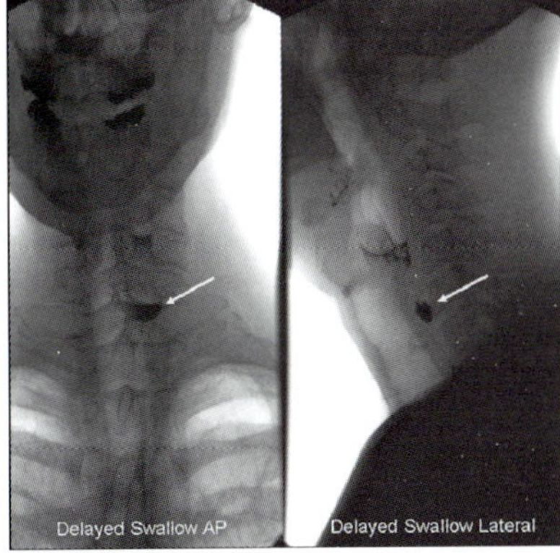

Figure 31.

Describe what you see and read on

The image obtained immediately after the initial swallow demonstrates an outpouching in the midline and posterior to the esophagus, measuring 18mm in the transverse plane by 6mm in the anteroposterior plane. These findings are suggestive of Zenker's diverticulum (white arrow). The initial swallow did not demonstrate the diverticulum as the barium was superimposed over it.

A small percentage of patients with Zenker's diverticulum have a second lesion more inferiorly, but no other lesions were seen in this patient.

What is the next step?

The main risks involved with Zenker's diverticulum include aspiration pneumonias and an enlarging diverticulum causing esophageal obstruction. Given the patient is symptomatic and having trouble with his medications, he will benefit from surgical treatment. Surgical options include:

- Excision of the diverticulum in one step.
- A two-stage operation, with mobilization of the diverticulum and excision at a later stage when granulation tissue has formed around the diverticulum.
- Cricopharyngeal myotomy leaving the diverticulum.
- Cricopharyngeal myotomy with diverticulectomy or diverticulopexy.

Currently, the most common method is to perform a transoral, stapled, cricopharyngeal muscle myotomy with a linear cutting stapler (the third option above). The diverticulum is a pouch that forms posterior to the upper esophageal sphincter (the cricopharyngeus muscle). Food catches here rather than entering the esophagus through the upper sphincter. Placing one arm of a stapler in the diverticulum and the other in the true lumen of the esophagus and firing the cutting stapler serves to transect the cricopharyngeus, thus connecting the diverticulum to the true lumen. The staples provide hemostasis and prevent perforation into the upper mediastinum. Similar endoscopic approaches exist, in which the septum between the diverticulum and the esophageal lumen (the circular cricopharyngeus muscle) is transected endoscopically using a needle knife or hook cautery.

Clinical pearls

- Patients with upper esophageal diverticula present with symptoms of dysphagia, food getting stuck, regurgitation of food, and even halitosis. Less fortunate patients can present with obstruction and recurrent aspiration pneumonia. Diagnosis is made with a barium swallow or endoscopy, and treatment is surgical.
- Zenker's diverticula arise because of a defect in the muscular wall of the hypopharynx. This can be caused by high pressures from a bolus of food during swallowing, or resistance of swallowing from abnormalities of the upper esophageal sphincter.
- Patients who have this diverticulum but have not been diagnosed carry an increased risk of perforation when a nasogastric tube or endoscope is passed.

Impress your attending

What are the various locations of the different esophageal diverticula?

- Zenker's diverticula: posterior to the upper esophageal sphincter.
- Traction diverticula: in the middle of the esophagus.
- Epiphrenic diverticula: just above the lower esophageal sphincter.
- Killian-Jamieson diverticula: very similar to a Zenker's diverticulum, but lateral to the upper esophageal sphincter rather than posterior.

What makes up Killian's triangle?

This is a triangular area in the cervical esophagus made up by the oblique fibers of the inferior constrictor muscle of the pharynx and the transverse fibers of the cricopharyngeus muscle.

Case 13

A 53-year-old man presents to his primary-care physician's office with a complaint of chest pain. He was seen 2 weeks ago by a nurse practitioner. Given his cardiac risk factors, which include hypercholesterolemia, smoking, and a family history of heart disease, a cardiac work-up was ordered. He returns today for the results, and also because of persistent symptoms. Review of the medical record shows the patient underwent an EKG, which demonstrated normal sinus rhythm, and an exercise treadmill stress test, which was also normal.

The patient says his symptoms have progressed. He describes his pain as a squeezing sensation in the substernal region. Eating aggravates the pain, and the pain he experiences varies in intensity. He says he has been having difficulty with solids and liquids for at least a month now. He feels that food gets stuck in his throat and at times regurgitates into his mouth, occurring mostly with liquids. Food eventually passes down into his stomach. He has had no weight loss, and has never experienced these symptoms before. He does not complain of a sour taste in the back of his throat and does not have a hoarse voice.

What is your differential diagnosis?

The differential diagnosis includes esophageal spasm, nutcracker esophagus, and gastroesophageal reflux disease.

Physical examination

Vitals Temperature 98.6°F, HR 80 bpm, BP 120/74mmHg, oxygen saturation 99% on RA.

GEN No obvious distress.

HEENT Moist mucous membranes. No scleral icterus. No lymphadenopathy.

CVS Normal S1, S2. No murmurs, rubs, or gallops.

RESP Clear to auscultation.

ABD Soft and non-tender. No rigidity, guarding, or rebound tenderness. Bowel sounds are present. Rectal examination deferred. Having the patient drink water does not reproduce the symptoms.

EXT No edema.

MSK Palpation over the chest wall does not reproduce symptoms.

Does this narrow your differential diagnosis?

Not significantly. The physical examination does not contribute much, but the history points toward a diagnosis of an esophageal motility disorder.

What diagnostic test will you order?

A barium swallow (esophagram).

This examination will evaluate the cervical, mid, and distal esophagus. This is different from a modified barium swallow/cine with speech therapy examination, which evaluates the swallowing mechanism with various food consistencies and does not evaluate the esophagus.

What blood test(s) will you order?

No blood test is needed. The patient's weight is steady, therefore checking the albumin level to assess his nutritional status is not indicated at this time. A CBC might be helpful to look for anemia. Cancers of the GI tract often bleed, so anemia might indicate a neoplasm as the source of his dysphagia.

The next step is to explain your differential diagnosis to the patient, and schedule the patient for follow-up within 2-3 days of completion of the study.

Imaging

The patient obtains his barium swallow (Figures 32 and 33).

Describe what you see and read on

Figure 32 shows an upright image of the patient's lower third of the esophagus opacified with thin liquid barium. Esophageal contractions are seen in the more mid to distal portion (white arrows). A 2cm hiatal hernia is seen distally (black arrow). There is no stricture or compression of the esophagus. Figure 33 shows a drinking film in the right anterior oblique projection, which shows a smooth esophagus demonstrating no strictures, webs, or abnormal impressions.

The radiology report also states the patient's chest pain was reproduced during the contractions. The contractions in fact were described as tertiary in nature, suggestive of esophageal spasm.

The patient returns to the clinic 2 days after his examination. How will you manage him?

A number of different therapies can be used to manage esophageal spasm. The first step is to treat this patient's symptoms. Options include nitrates or anti-cholinergics such as hyoscyamine, which can be taken prior to a meal.

If the symptoms were predominantly causing chest pain then treatment options would include phosphodiesterase inhibitors or calcium-channel blockers such as diltiazem.

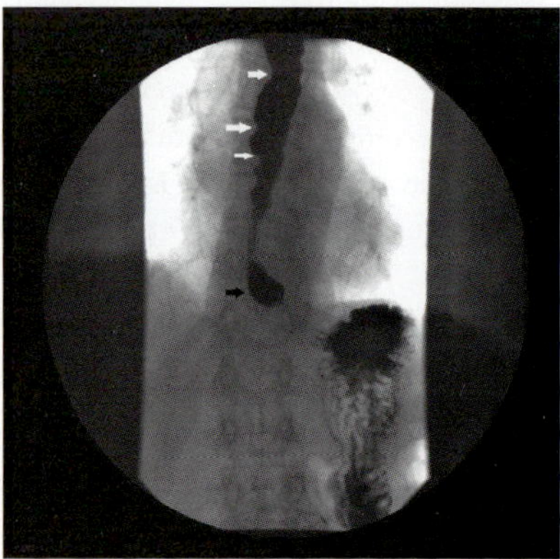

Figure 32.

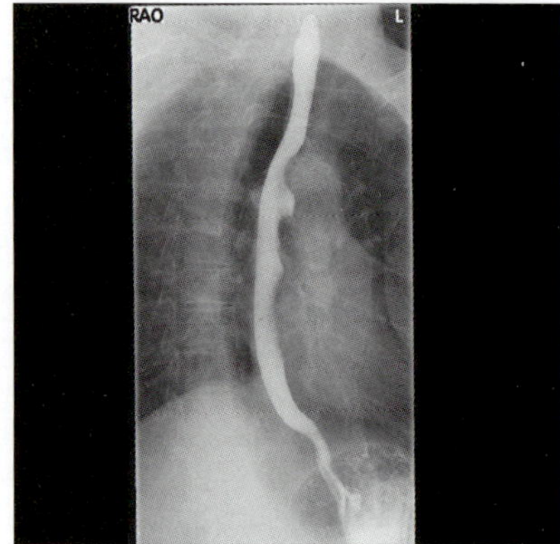

Figure 33.

This patient was given a trial of an anti-cholinergic agent, which greatly improved his symptoms.

Clinical pearls

- Esophageal spasms can present with non-specific chest pain caused by motility problems.
- Although this diagnosis is included in the differential diagnosis for chest pain, it is a rare cause.
- Diagnosis can be made with a barium swallow or esophageal manometry.

Impress your attending

How do you perform esophageal manometry?

Esophageal manometry is the measurement of intraluminal pressure within the esophagus during rest and during 10 sips of water. The patient should be nil by mouth for approximately 8 hours. First, a local anesthetic gel is placed in one nostril, which also provides lubrication. A manometry probe is then inserted into the nostril and passed into the esophagus as the patient swallows. The probe is connected to the manometer, which records pressure readings at different locations during rest and during swallows.

What findings on esophageal manometry suggest esophageal spasms?

The hallmark finding is excessive simultaneous contractions in the distal esophagus more than 20% of the time. High-amplitude, prolonged contractions can also be seen specifically with esophageal spasms.

Case 14

A 19-year-old man presents to the emergency room with abdominal pain. The pain began 1 day prior and is mostly located in the epigastric region. He describes it as sharp and constant. It radiates to the right upper quadrant and at times he feels it is all over his abdomen. He gives the pain a 10/10 in severity. Lying still relieves the pain, while moving around aggravates it. Associated symptoms include vomiting and loss of appetite. The patient has no diarrhea and no urinary symptoms. He is passing flatus.

The patient says he had this pain a few months ago, but it was not as severe and subsided on its own. None of his contacts are unwell. He traveled to Turkey 1 month ago to visit his parents. The patient says he stopped taking a medication his mother used to give him after he moved to the USA 4 years ago. He does not know the name of this medication or what it was for. He had abdominal surgery as a child, but again does not know what it was for. He has no other past medical history, denies alcohol or recreational drug use, and has no drug allergies. He is a full-time college student. He was hit in the abdomen when he missed a ground ball during baseball practice 2 weeks ago.

What is your differential diagnosis?

The differential diagnosis includes hepatitis, pancreatitis, ulcer disease, and cholecystitis.

Physical examination

Vitals Temperature 101.5°F, HR 110 bpm, BP 100/60mmHg, respiratory rate 20 breaths per minute, oxygen saturation 98% on RA.

GEN Does not look distressed.

HEENT Moist mucous membranes. No scleral icterus. No lymphadenopathy.

CVS Tachycardic. Normal S1, S2. No murmurs, rubs, or gallops.

RESP Normal chest expansion. Clear to auscultation.

ABD A well-healed laparotomy scar is noted. The abdomen is diffusely tender, especially in the epigastric region. Rigidity and guarding are present. Bowel sounds are faint. Rectal examination reveals an empty vault with guaiac-negative stool.

EXT There is an erythematous, tender, raised lesion over the right medial ankle measuring 5 x 3cm with sharp, well-defined borders.

Does the physical examination change the differential diagnosis?

Yes. The physical examination findings add a diagnosis to the differential that is a surgical emergency.

While the surgical team is mobilized to assess the patient, which blood tests should be ordered?

CBC	WBC	18 x 10^3/μL with a left shift
	Hemoglobin	14.3g/dL
	Hematocrit	41%
	Platelets	240 x 10^3/μL
CHEM-7	Na	141mEq/L
	K	3.1mEq/L
	Cl	103mEq/L
	Bicarbonate	23mEq/L
	BUN	18mg/dL
	Creatinine	1.0mg/dL
	Glucose	92mg/dL
LFTs	AST	23 units/L
	ALT	25 units/L
	Alkaline phosphatase	56 units/L
Lipase		20 units/L
ESR		56mm/h

What is the rationale for abdominal imaging as opposed to going straight to the operating room?

The patient has had a laparotomy in the past and it would therefore be beneficial to know his abdominal anatomy prior to surgical exploration. Imaging may even provide a diagnosis. In any other situation, including a more unstable patient, bypassing imaging and going straight to the operating room decreases mortality.

The images obtained from a similar patient are shown in Figures 34 and 35.

Describe what you see and read on

Limited axial and coronal images through the mid-abdomen demonstrate mildly dilated, fluid-filled proximal small-bowel loops up to 4cm (white arrows), with normal-appearing distal small bowel (Figure 34, yellow arrow) and colon. There is no discrete transition point. There is no free air or suggestion of a perforated viscus.

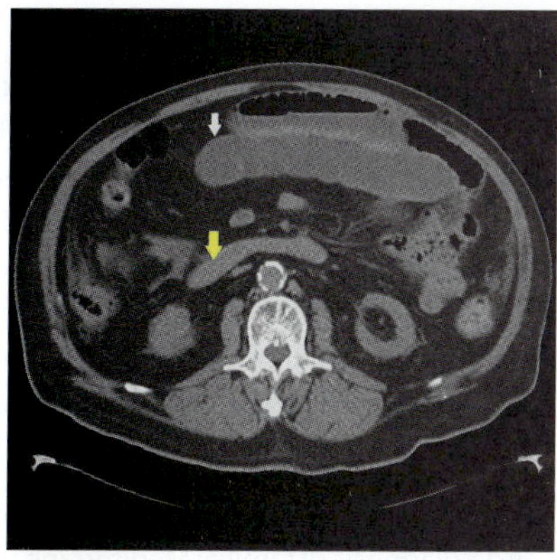

Figure 34.

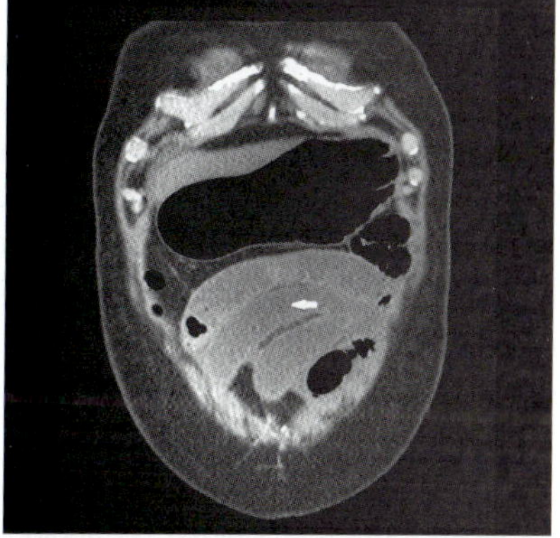

Figure 35.

Given the finding of an ileus, the surgical team decides there is no surgical emergency and an alternative diagnosis should be sought.

What is the next step?

The next step is to ensure the patient has adequate IV access, and provide IV pain control and fluids. The patient must remain nil by mouth.

An ileus is a highly unlikely cause of the physical examination findings. The CT scan essentially rules out all of the other disease processes that were entertained. At this point, a bright clinician will be able to make this diagnosis by putting together key information from the history and recognizing the missing data the patient cannot provide.

The patient is of Mediterranean descent, and a diagnosis of familial Mediterranean fever fits his clinical symptoms. This condition is characterized by paroxysmal episodes of fever and serosal inflammation with abdominal pain that subsides on its own over the course of 4 days. The ileus was most likely caused by the serosal inflammation (not shown on this CT scan), and will be treated with conservative therapy.

The patient most likely presented to the hospital with similar symptoms when he was much younger and had a laparotomy that yielded no findings. It is likely he was taking colchicine as a preventative therapy while he lived in Turkey and did not continue it after he moved to the USA.

Clinical pearls

- Familial Mediterranean fever is an autosomal recessive disorder characterized by paroxysmal episodes of fever and serosal inflammation leading to abdominal pain. Patients have an elevated WBC and acute-phase reactants.
- Patients are usually of Mediterranean descent.
- Monoarthritis can also be present. An absence of alternative causes of arthritis is part of the diagnostic criteria.
- Colchicine is the mainstay of preventative therapy.

Impress your attending

How would you treat the erythematous lesion on this patient's right ankle?

Patients with familial Mediterranean fever, especially those from the Eastern Mediterranean, can also develop erysipelas-like skin lesions. The lesion will regress spontaneously. There is no need for antibiotics.

Case 15

A 63-year-old woman presents to her primary-care physician for her yearly physical. She has no trouble with her day-to-day activities. Her weight is steady, and she does not feel fatigued at all. Her arthritis of the knees does not generally bother her, and if needed she takes ibuprofen. Overall, she feels quite well. Her medical history includes type 2 diabetes, which is controlled with metformin. Her last HbA1c level was 6.5%. She is up to date with her mammograms, colorectal cancer screening, and pap smears.

Physical examination

Vitals Temperature 97.8°F, HR 74 bpm, BP 120/80mmHg, oxygen saturation 99% on RA.

GEN No obvious distress. Looks healthy.

HEENT Moist mucous membranes. No scleral icterus. No lymphadenopathy.

CVS Normal S1, S2. No murmurs, rubs, or gallops.

RESP Clear to auscultation.

ABD Soft and non-tender. There is a palpable firm mass in the right mid-clavicular line, below the costal margin, noticeable only on deep palpation. The liver, by palpation and percussion, measures 15cm. No splenomegaly. No rigidity, guarding, or rebound tenderness. Bowel sounds are normal. Rectal examination reveals guaiac-negative stool.

EXT No clubbing or edema.

What is your differential diagnosis?

The physical examination leads the clinician toward pathology in the hepatobiliary region. The patient's abdomen is not tender on examination and offers no signs or symptoms of malignancy. The differential diagnosis at this point would include a mass arising off the inferior margin of the liver or from the gallbladder.

What imaging test will you order?

Portable ultrasound is becoming readily available in clinician offices. Starting with an ultrasound, especially for a palpable mass in the right upper quadrant, is the most cost-effective plan for working up this patient. The images obtained are shown in Figures 36 and 37.

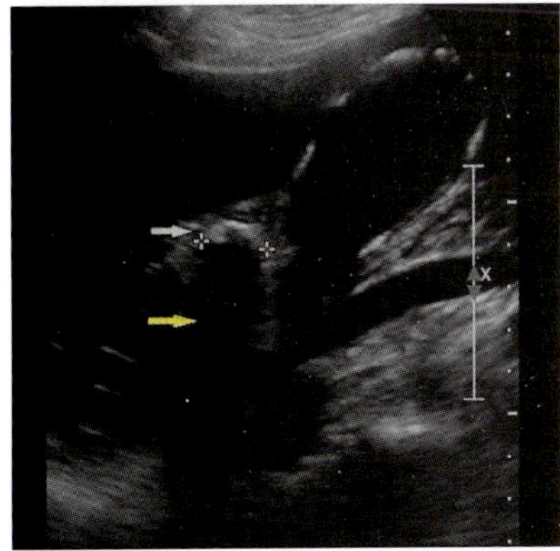

Figure 36.

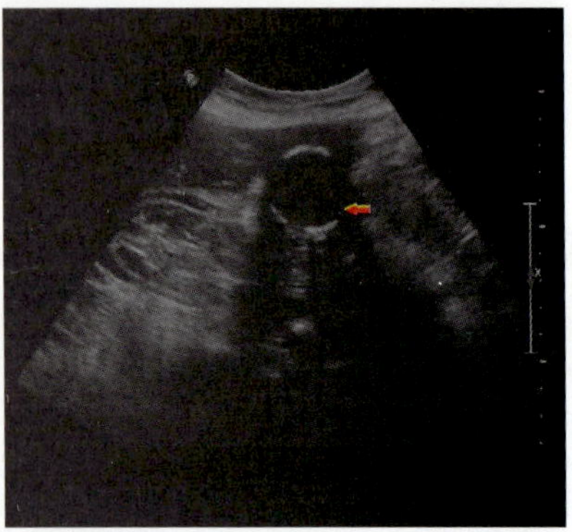

Figure 37.

Describe what you see and read on

Transverse (Figure 36) and sagittal (Figure 37) images obtained from a portable ultrasound of the right upper quadrant show hyperechoic material in the wall of the gallbladder. Echogenic material is seen in the lumen in the dependent portion, most likely representing minimal sludge (red arrow). A 1cm echogenic focus (white arrow) with posterior acoustic shadowing (yellow arrow) is identified in the neck of the gallbladder, representing a gallstone or dense calcification of the wall. There is no pericholecystic fluid. The gallbladder wall is difficult to measure, but appears to be slightly larger than 3mm.

These findings are consistent with a porcelain gallbladder with cholelithiasis.

What is the next step?

The next step is to go back to the history and obtain more information from the patient. Porcelain gallbladder is an uncommon manifestation of chronic cholecystitis, and asking specific questions related to the biliary system would therefore be useful. At this point the patient is asymptomatic, which is very common with this entity.

The patient will need to be referred to a surgeon to have the gallbladder removed. Porcelain gallbladder is associated with adenocarcinoma of the gallbladder in approximately 12-60% of cases.

What blood test(s) will you order before surgical referral?

A CBC will check for anemia, which can be associated with malignancy.

CBC	**WBC**	7.5 x 10^3/μL
	Hemoglobin	14.2g/dL
	Hematocrit	41%
	Platelets	270 x 10^3/μL

Clinical pearls

- Porcelain gallbladder is often incidentally found on routine imaging (i.e., a plain film of the abdomen, abdominal CT scan, or ultrasound).
- The incidence is only 0.06%. Most patients are asymptomatic, but this condition can also present as right upper quadrant pain or, rarely, a palpable mass.
- Porcelain gallbladder is associated with an increased risk of adenocarcinoma. Surgical removal is therefore advised, even in asymptomatic patients.

Impress your attending

Name two ultrasound patterns used to characterize porcelain gallbladders

- Complete type: the gallbladder wall is completely replaced by dense calcification, in that there is a semilunar appearance with dense posterior acoustic shadowing.

- Incomplete type: the gallbladder wall is incompletely calcified. This has a milder clinical course than the complete type. Acoustic shadowing is still seen.

Case 16

A 46-year-old woman presents to the emergency room with abdominal pain. The pain began about 25 minutes after eating dinner. It is located in the epigastric region. She describes it as a steady pain that radiates to her back and right shoulder. She rates it 8/10 in intensity. The pain is worse on deep inspiration. Associated symptoms include nausea, vomiting, and fever. She did not notice blood in her emesis.

The patient says she had a milder episode of this pain years ago, but that it went away on its own. She is not taking any prescription medications or over-the-counter drugs such as aspirin or NSAIDs. She has not traveled recently, and has no allergies. The patient usually lives an active lifestyle, playing squash a few times a week. There are no cardiac or respiratory issues in her review of symptoms.

What is your differential diagnosis?

The differential diagnosis includes acute cholecystitis, acute pancreatitis, symptomatic cholelithiasis, peptic ulcer disease, and gastritis.

Physical examination

Vitals Temperature 102.5°F, HR 108 bpm, BP 110/60mmHg, oxygen saturation 98% on RA.

GEN Appears unwell.

HEENT No scleral icterus or lymphadenopathy.

CVS Tachycardic. Normal S1, S2. No murmurs, rubs, or gallops.

RESP Decreased breath sounds at the right base.

ABD Tender and voluntary guarding. Palpation just below the liver margin causes discomfort and inspiratory arrest. Bowel sounds are normal. Rectal examination reveals an empty vault.

EXT No edema.

Does this alter your differential diagnosis?

Yes, it does. This patient has a positive Murphy's sign, so cholecystitis is the most likely diagnosis.

What blood test(s) will you order?

CBC	WBC	17 x 10^3/μL
	Hemoglobin	14g/dL
	Hematocrit	41.7%
	Platelets	340 x 10^3/μL
CHEM-7	Na	140mEq/L
	K	3.6mEq/L
	Cl	101mEq/L
	Bicarbonate	24mEq/L
	BUN	16mg/dL
	Creatinine	1.1mg/dL
	Glucose	101mg/dL
LFTs	AST	26 units/L

ALT	90 units/L
Alkaline phosphatase	161 units/L
Total bilirubin	1.6mg/dL

What do these laboratory data suggest?

The elevated WBC suggests an infection. A differential count would show increased bands (also known as a left shift). These are the expected laboratory findings in uncomplicated cholecystitis.

The patient's laboratory values also suggest an early cholestatic process. The alkaline phosphatase and ALT levels are elevated, suggesting a possible component of common bile duct obstruction. Mild kidney injury also appears to be present, but this would need to be compared to prior creatinine levels.

What imaging test will you order?

The next step is to obtain an ultrasound of the abdomen, looking specifically at the right upper quadrant (Figures 38 and 39).

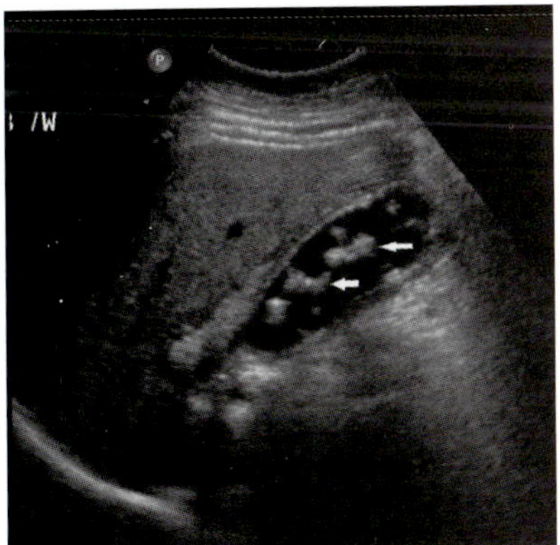

Figure 38.

Describe what you see and read on

The ultrasound shows a gallbladder in the transverse (Figure 38) and sagittal (Figure 39) views. Numerous echogenic foci are identified within the lumen of the gallbladder, representing gallstones (white arrows). A thickened gallbladder wall (red arrow) and fluid adjacent to the wall (yellow arrow) are also seen.

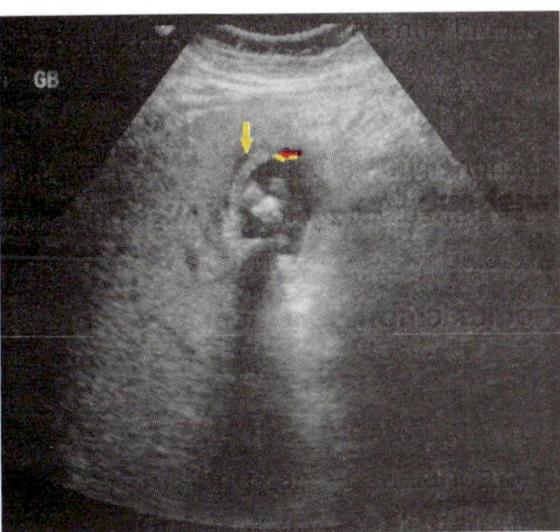

Figure 39.

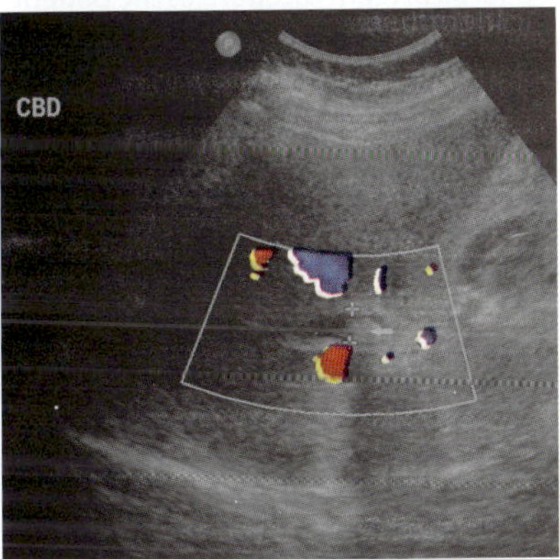

Figure 40.

A further image is obtained (Figure 40).

Describe what you see and read on

This is a single image of the common bile duct in the sagittal view (between the calipers), showing an echogenic focus with posterior acoustic shadowing representing a stone (white arrow) in a dilated common bile duct. Color Doppler interrogation demonstrates this is not a vascular structure.

The next step is to admit the patient, keep her nil by mouth, start IV fluids, and call for an admission to the surgical service.

What is the diagnosis, and how will you proceed?

The constellation of findings of cholelithiasis, a thick gallbladder wall, and pericholecystic fluid is most often diagnostic of acute cholecystitis. The positive Murphy's sign elicited on physical examination adds to the positive predictive value of this being the diagnosis. The stone in the common bile duct also gives the patient a diagnosis of choledocholithiasis.

Management

The surgical team categorizes the patient as an ASA 1, which allows her to undergo an early cholecystectomy. Inflammation tends to get worse by 72 hours from the onset of symptoms. While waiting for surgery, pain control is indicated and ketorolac is given. Narcotics can cause sphincter of Oddi spasm, which in theory could make the obstructive process in the common bile duct worse. However, it is common practice to use narcotic analgesia in this setting and it does not appear to be harmful. Given the patient's fever and leukocytosis, broad-spectrum antibiotics are also indicated, such as piperacillin-tazobactam, cefotetan, ampicillin-sulbactam, or cefoxitin. The patient will have a cholecystectomy during the current hospitalization.

Clinical pearls

- Acute cholecystitis is a syndrome of abdominal pain, low-grade liver enzyme abnormality, and fever caused by inflammation of the gallbladder. In most cases, it is caused by gallstones.
- Gallbladder pain can present in the right upper quadrant or epigastric region, and sometimes radiates to the right scapula.
- Although cholecystitis is not always infectious in origin, broad-spectrum antibiotics are indicated while awaiting surgical consultation.
- Treatment is usually surgical, with either immediate or delayed cholecystectomy based on surgical risk.
- Untreated cholecystitis may abate on its own in about a week.

Impress your attending

What are the complications of cholecystitis?

Complications include gangrene, perforation, cholecystoenteric fistula, gallstone ileus, and septic shock leading to death.

Case 17

Earlier in the afternoon, a 42-year-old man ate lunch and then went for a swim. While swimming, he developed abdominal pain. The pain failed to subside and he presented to the emergency room a few hours later. The pain is located in the lower abdomen and just slightly to the right of the midline and does not radiate anywhere. He describes it as a constant pain that is 7/10 in severity. There are no specific aggravating or relieving factors. Although it has only been a few hours, he feels he has had no change in his appetite. He does not have bowel symptoms, nausea, or vomiting. His entire family ate the same food, which was fresh, for lunch and no-one has similar symptoms. The patient just wants to lie still.

What is your differential diagnosis?

The differential diagnosis includes diverticulitis, appendicitis, abdominal muscle strain, and early gastroenteritis.

Physical examination

Vitals Afebrile, HR 92 bpm, BP 130/76mmHg, oxygen saturation 99% on RA.

GEN Does not appear ill.

Hands No clubbing. No signs of chronic liver disease.

HEENT No scleral icterus or pale conjunctivae.

CVS Normal S1, S2. No murmurs, rubs, or gallops.

RESP Clear to auscultation.

ABD Tenderness in the right lower quadrant. No rebound tenderness or rigidity. Bowel sounds are normal. Rectal examination reveals guaiac-negative stool.

EXT No edema.

What initial blood test(s) will you order?

CBC	WBC	8.5 x 10^3/μL
	Hemoglobin	14.7g/dL
	Hematocrit	40.7%
	Platelets	330 x 10^3/μL
ESR		28mm/h

What other blood tests will you order?

CHEM-7, LFTs, lipase.

All are within normal limits.

The patient's blood panel is not revealing. The ESR is slightly elevated, but this is a non-specific finding.

The patient continues to experience severe pain. IV analgesics are administered with some relief. The physician next orders a CT scan of the abdomen and pelvis (Figures 41 and 42).

Describe what you see and read on

In the axial (Figure 41) and coronal (Figure 42) images, contrast is seen extending as far as the sigmoid colon.

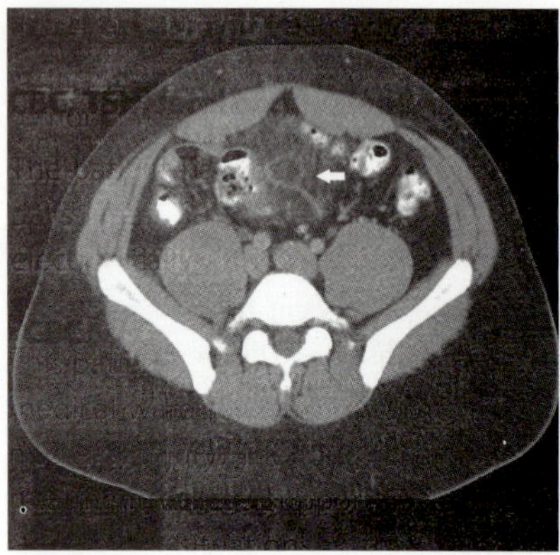

Figure 41.

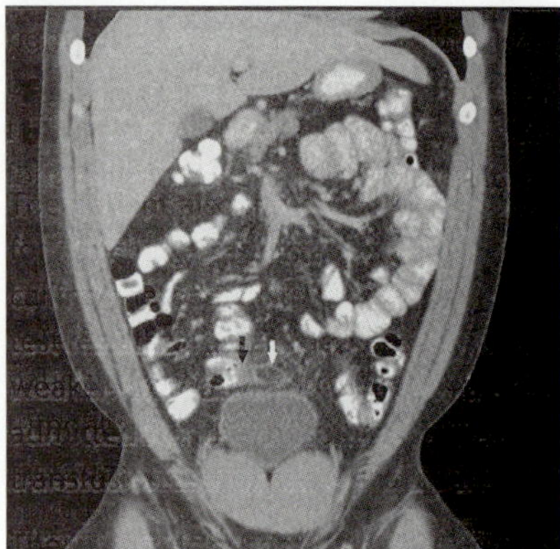

Figure 42.

The small bowel is normal in size and caliber. The ascending, transverse, and descending colon are unremarkable. There is asymmetric thickening of the sigmoid colon (black arrow) secondary to inflammation in the adjacent fat (white arrows) in the midline in the supravesicular region. The bladder wall appears normal. No diverticula are identified. No adjacent pericolonic fluid collections are seen. The findings are consistent with epiploic appendagitis.

Management

Epiploic appendagitis is a benign condition that does not require hospitalization. The patient will need NSAIDs such as ibuprofen 600mg three times a day for up to a week, along with other pain-control medication if needed. The patient should be advised to return to the emergency room or his primary-care physician if his symptoms do not improve in the next few days.

Clinical pearls

- Epiploic appendages are fat-filled outpouchings that are present all over the colon.
- Epiploic appendagitis occurs when there is torsion of the supplying vessel to the appendage.
- The symptoms often mimic diverticulitis, appendicitis, or even an acute abdomen.
- The key difference is the lack of a high white cell count or fever.

Impress your attending

Although uncommon, what are some possible complications of epiploic appendagitis?

- Abscess formation.
- Adherence to the abdominal wall or other abdominal organs, which can lead to intestinal obstruction or intussusception.

Case 18

A 24-year-old man presents to the emergency department with abdominal pain. The pain is diffuse and crampy in nature. It is constant and he rates it 6/10 in severity. It began about 48 hours prior to presentation and has not subsided. The pain does not radiate anywhere. There are no specific aggravating or relieving factors. The patient says he has had non-bloody diarrhea for the past week, and has noticed his stools floating more. His appetite has decreased and he has experienced 10 lbs of weight loss. He has also felt feverish off and on, but has not taken his temperature. As a result of the symptoms, the patient has become quite fatigued.

None of his contacts are unwell, and he and his family have eaten the same foods all week. He has not traveled recently. Review of his systems does not demonstrate rheumatologic or other constitutional symptoms. He has never experienced symptoms like this before. The patient smokes a pack of cigarettes a day.

What is your differential diagnosis?

The differential diagnosis includes inflammatory bowel disease, infectious colitis, and irritable bowel syndrome.

Physical examination

Vitals	Temperature 101.7°F, HR 98 bpm, BP 100/70mmHg, oxygen saturation 99% on RA.
GEN	Appears unwell.
Hands	Decreased skin turgor. Clubbing.
H+N	No scleral icterus and dry mucous membranes.
CVS	Normal S1, S2. No murmurs, rubs, or gallops.
RESP	Clear to auscultation.
ABD	Slightly tender but soft. No rigidity, guarding, or rebound tenderness. Bowel sounds are present. Rectal examination reveals an empty vault.
EXT	No edema.

What blood test(s) will you order?

CBC	WBC	14 x $10^3/\mu L$ with no left shift
	Hemoglobin	12.8g/dL
	Hematocrit	37.3%
	Platelets	321 x $10^3/\mu L$

What other blood test(s) will you order?

CHEM-7, ESR, CRP, serum iron, and vitamin B12 levels.

CHEM-7	Na	139mEq/L
	K	3.1mEq/L
	Cl	103mEq/L
	Bicarbonate	25mEq/L
	BUN	20mg/dL

	Creatinine	1.3mg/dL
	Glucose	101mg/dL
ESR and CRP		Slightly
Iron studies and vitamin B12		Not available at this time

What do these laboratory data suggest?

The patient has an inflammatory process. WBC, ESR, and CRP can be elevated during the acute phase of inflammation. Given the extensive diarrhea along with the physical findings, the patient has renal injury most likely secondary to dehydration.

What is the next step?

The patient already has low BP and an elevated creatinine level, so it is imperative to start IV fluids. It is also important to rule out infectious diarrhea with a stool sample.

What imaging test will you order?

A CT scan of the abdomen and pelvis with oral and IV contrast (Figures 43 and 44) should be considered once the acute kidney injury has been addressed.

Describe what you see and read on

The images shown are an axial (Figure 43) and coronal (Figure 44) view of the abdomen with oral and IV contrast. The stomach is unremarkable. Distended loops of the small bowel are not seen. There is marked wall thickening with a small amount of adjacent fluid and fat stranding at the terminal ileum (white arrow). The colon is of normal caliber. The cecum and right colon are filled with fluid (black arrow). The appendix is normal (not shown). No adenopathy is identified.

The differential diagnosis for these findings includes an inflammatory process such as Crohn's disease, or an infectious process such as bacterial enteritis as from *Campylobacter jejuni,* Salmonella species, or *Escherichia coli.* Although less likely, an ischemic etiology is possible.

What is the next step?

Given how unwell the patient appears, he should be admitted for the treatment of Crohn's disease. He should be sent to the regular medical ward and started on treatment.

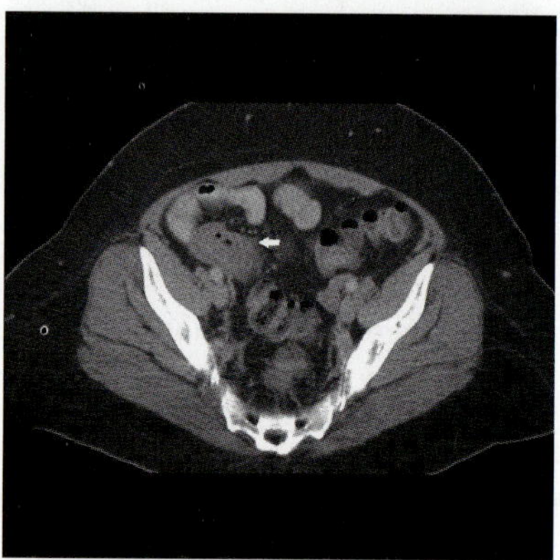

Figure 43.

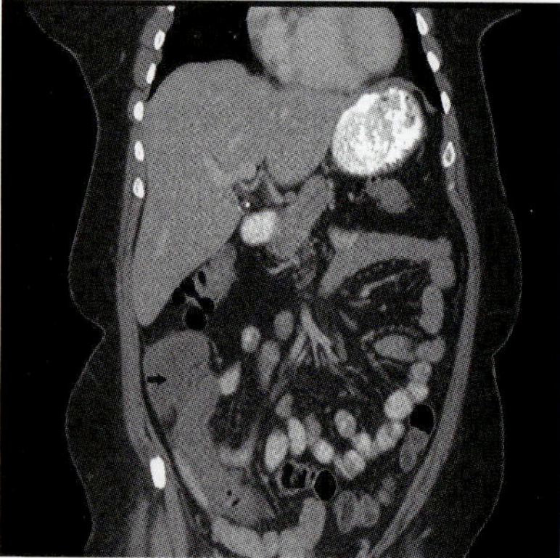

Figure 44.

Given the fact his disease appears specific to the ileum, he should be started on an

IV steroid such as methylprednisolone. When he improves he can be switched to an oral corticosteroid such as budesonide or prednisone. Gastroenterology consultation should be obtained for colonoscopy with biopsy of the terminal ileum, and to institute more advanced levels of therapy (e.g., azathioprine, mercaptopurine, infliximab, adalimumab).

A classic endoscopic image of a colon in a patient with Crohn's disease is shown in Figure 45.

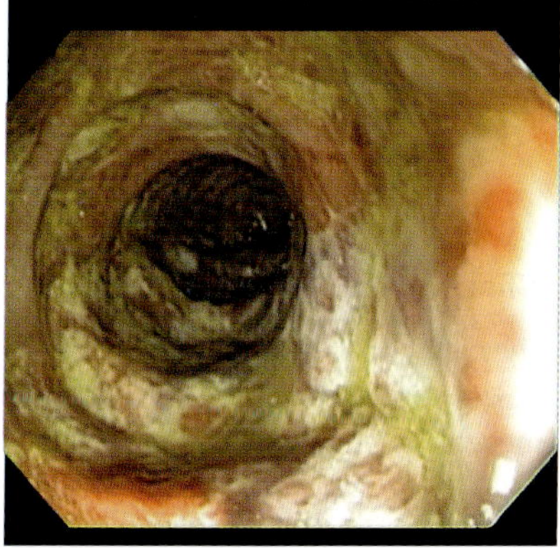

Figure 45.

Although this is not the same patient, the endoscopic picture shown in Figure 45 demonstrates the characteristic findings seen in Crohn's colitis, which include friability (i.e., easy bleeding when touched), ulceration, erythema, and edema.

Clinical pearls

- Crohn's disease is protean in its presenting features, but often presents with crampy abdominal pain and diarrhea. Fatigue is common.
- Most patients are first diagnosed between the ages of 20 and 30 years.
- Extraintestinal manifestations of Crohn's disease include arthritis, pyoderma gangrenosum, uveitis, primary sclerosing cholangitis, thromboembolism secondary to hypercoagulability, renal stones, vitamin B12 deficiency, and fistula formation.

Impress your attending

What kind of renal stones do patients with Crohn's disease experience?

Calcium oxalate. This is because there is excessive GI absorption of oxalate, leading to hyperoxaluria. In turn, the intestinal fat binds dietary calcium, which is then not available to bind to oxalate as it normally does.

How is the distribution of Crohn's disease different from that of ulcerative colitis?

Crohn's disease has skip lesions and can occur anywhere in the GI tract, sparing the rectum. Ulcerative colitis is continuous from the rectum and extends proximally.

Fact: smoking is a risk factor for Crohn's disease. This is not the case for ulcerative colitis.

What is indeterminate colitis?

Crohn's colitis is sometimes indistinguishable from ulcerative colitis, both endoscopically and histologically. If there are not enough clues in the history and presentation to determine whether a patient has Crohn's or ulcerative colitis, then the patient may be designated as having 'indeterminate colitis.' Since the treatments for ulcerative colitis and Crohn's vary significantly, a designation of indeterminate colitis can pose a problem when developing a management plan.

Case 19

A 52-year-old man who is receiving anticoagulation for atrial fibrillation presents to the emergency room with abdominal pain. His pain is located slightly to the left of the midline, predominantly in the epigastric region. He describes the pain as a dull ache that began 2 hours ago while watching television. The pain does not radiate anywhere. He rates it 5/10 in intensity. There are no specific aggravating or relieving factors. The patient says he has experienced this pain off and on for the past year, but it has never lasted this long. He denies other symptoms such as nausea, vomiting, or diarrhea.

The patient has not exerted himself in any way, other than his usual activities of daily living. He does not feel feverish and apart from the abdominal pain, has no other symptoms. He says he has not passed gas in the past couple of hours, but that is his norm. The patient has not been constipated.

Physical examination

Vitals Temperature 98.5°F, HR 96 bpm, BP 120/60mmHg, oxygen saturation 98% on RA.

GEN No apparent distress.

HEENT No scleral icterus or lymphadenopathy.

CVS Tachycardic. Normal S1, S2. No murmurs, rubs, or gallops.

RESP Normal chest expansion and clear to auscultation.

ABD The abdomen is tender slightly to the left of the midline in the epigastric region. There is a palpable mass that is deep and ovoid in shape, measuring up to 4cm. There is no rigidity or guarding. Bowel sounds are slightly hyperactive. The rectal vault is full of stool, which is guaiac-negative.

EXT No edema.

What is your differential diagnosis?

The differential diagnosis includes small-bowel obstruction, bowel ischemia, mesenteric adenitis, intussusception, gastric volvulus, and acute pancreatitis.

What blood test(s) will you order?

CBC	WBC	7 x 10^3/μL
	Hemoglobin	14g/dL
	Hematocrit	41.1%
	Platelets	350 x 10^3/μL
CHEM-7	Na	140mEq/L
	K	3.8mEq/L
	Cl	100mEq/L
	Bicarbonate	25mEq/L
	BUN	16mg/dL
	Creatinine	1.0mg/dL
	Glucose	94mg/dL
INR		2.3
Lactate		1.0mmol/L

What do these laboratory data suggest?

The pertinent findings in the laboratory data suggest that an embolus to the bowel causing infarction or ischemia is less likely because the patient has a therapeutic INR. The normal lactate level also argues against bowel infarction or ischemia. The remainder of the blood work does not suggest any other abnormality.

What imaging test will you order?

The next step is to obtain a CT scan of the abdomen and pelvis (Figures 46 and 47).

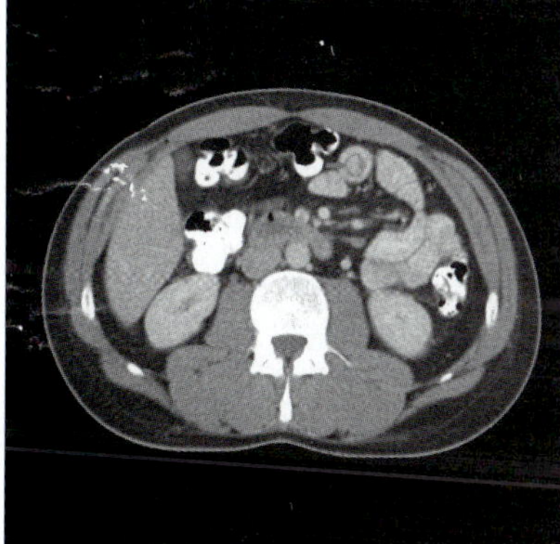

Figure 46.

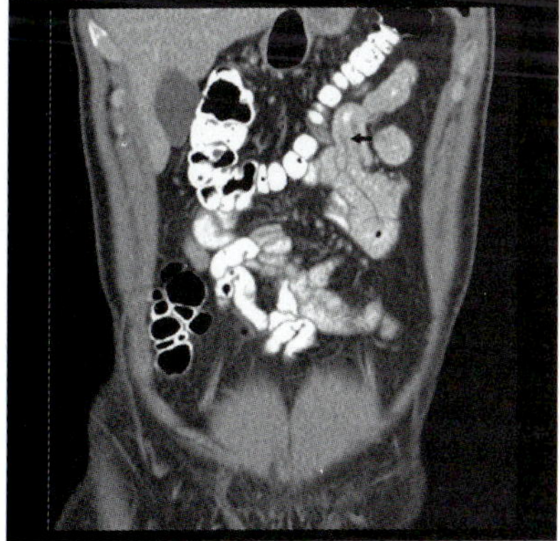

Figure 47.

Describe what you see and read on

Presented above are two images in the axial (Figure 46) and coronal (Figure 47) planes. The patient has been given both oral and IV contrast. In the proximal to mid-jejunum there is a loop of bowel with a hypodense rim (red arrow). Another soft-tissue structure within it most likely represents another loop of bowel (black arrow). This segment measures up to 3cm and is most representative of an enteroenteric intussusception. There is no adjacent inflammatory change in the mesentery. No adenopathy is identified.

Intussusception is a prolapse of the bowel that can lead to obstruction and eventually compromise the blood supply to the affected region. The lead point is often a site of malignancy in adults.

The next step is to obtain a surgical consultation to guide further management.

Management

Establishing IV access and pain control are the first priorities. Correcting electrolyte derangements is imperative. However, this patient has no electrolyte abnormalities. If the intussusception is larger than 3.5cm, then operative management is the treatment of choice, as there is often an underlying malignancy. However, non-operative management is preferred when the segment is shorter than 3.5cm, as intussusceptions of this length in adults are usually considered transient. This patient can be discharged from the emergency room and should follow-up with a surgeon as an outpatient. He should also be advised to return to the emergency room if his symptoms worsen or recur.

Two weeks later, the patient's primary-care physician orders a small-bowel study. It shows the following image (Figure 48).

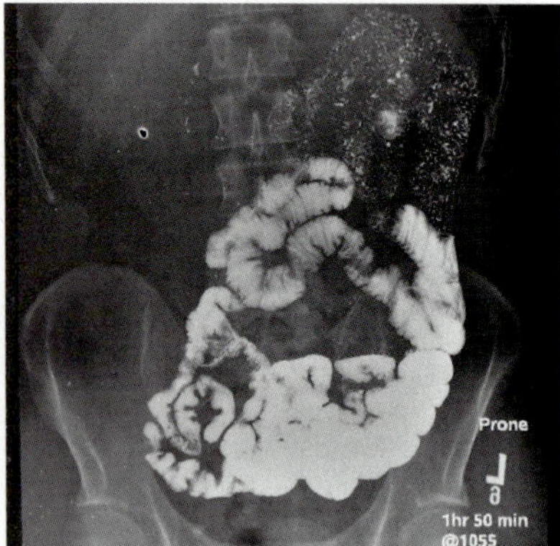

Figure 48.

Describe what you see and read on

There is no evidence of bowel malrotation. Transit time through the small intestine at this point is about 2 hours. Jejunal and ileal loops demonstrate a normal course and caliber without mucosal abnormality, fixed filling defect, stricture, or mass effect. There is no evidence of intussusception. The terminal ileum is not visible on this film.

This demonstrates the intussusception was a transient finding that has resolved.

Clinical pearls

- Intussusception is a rare finding in adults.
- Patients typically present with signs and symptoms of bowel obstruction.
- Management is based on the size:
  - conservative management is preferred if the segment is shorter than 3.5cm;
  - treatment is surgical if the segment is longer than 3.5cm.
- Electrolyte abnormalities should always be corrected.

Impress your attending

What are the different types of intussusceptions?

- Enteroenteric (small bowel).
- Colo-colonic (large bowel).
- Ileocolic (the terminal ileum protrudes into the ascending colon).
- Ileocecal (the ileocecal valve is the lead point into the cecum).

Case 20

A 47-year-old man presents to his primary-care physician complaining of dysphagia. He first started to notice the symptoms 2 years ago. At first the problem was only with solid food; however, over the past month he has begun to have trouble with liquids as well. He often feels fullness in the retrosternal region after a meal. He has also had difficulty with belching. He has lost about 10 lbs and attributes this to eating less. He often regurgitates food, especially at night, and it appears undigested. His wife complains about his bad breath and how he throws his shoulders back to get food down at times. There is no history of recent travel.

What is your differential diagnosis?

The differential diagnosis includes an esophageal motility disorder, esophageal stricture or ring, and esophageal malignancy.

Physical examination

Vitals Afebrile, HR 86 bpm, BP 110/78mmHg, oxygen saturation 99% on RA.

GEN Does not appear ill or cachectic.

Hands No clubbing.

HEENT No scleral icterus or pale conjunctivae. No adenopathy. No Virchow's node. No signs of raised jugular venous pressure. Halitosis is present.

CVS Normal S1, S2. No murmurs, rubs, or gallops.

RESP Minimal crackles at the bases.

ABD Soft and non-tender. No rigidity, guarding, or rebound tenderness. No organomegaly. Bowel sounds are normal.

EXT Trace edema at the ankles.

What blood test(s) will you order?

A CBC is ordered because anemia would suggest malignancy. However, the CBC is entirely normal.

Does your differential diagnosis change with the physical examination findings?

No. The examination does not change the differential diagnosis for the dysphagia. The examination does add an element of fluid overload with the crackles and the edema at the ankles. Further history clarifies the patient has experienced ankle swelling for years.

Imaging

The primary-care physician obtains a portable chest radiograph in the office (Figure 49).

Describe what you see and read on

The trachea is central. There are large pockets of encapsulated interlobar pleural effusion bilaterally, principally in the more superior aspect of the major fissures (black arrows). At least some free fluid also covers the diaphragm. There is mild prominence of central lung markings. In the base of the neck and upper mediastinum, there is evidence of marked gaseous distention of the esophagus with a diameter of at least 6cm (white arrows). Although this is an anteroposterior film the heart appears enlarged, consistent with cardiomegaly.

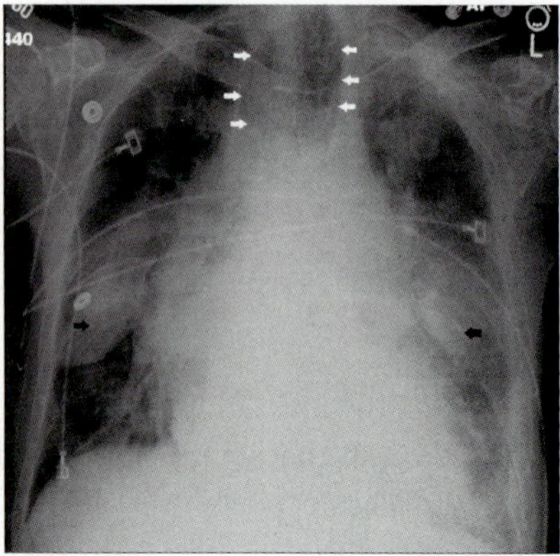

Figure 49.

Given the imaging findings, with a dilated esophagus and cardiomegaly, the primary-care physician further inquires whether the patient has ever traveled to South America. The patient says he was there 15 years ago. He now recalls being slightly ill after the trip, but then got better.

What blood test(s) will you order at this time?

Trypanosoma cruzi serologic testing.

The patient is also scheduled for a barium swallow study (Figure 50).

Describe what you see and read on

This is an anteroposterior fluoroscopic image using thin liquid barium. There is marked dilatation of the esophagus, particularly in the mid and distal portion (white arrows) with narrowing at the gastroesophageal junction. The narrowed segment forms after a short'bird's beak' appearance (black arrow). The narrowed segment measures 3cm (yellow arrow) in length. Filling defects are apparent in the esophagus, and most likely represent food particles within the dilated esophagus. Barium is seen entering the stomach. The rectangular opacity on the patient's left is the cup of barium he is holding.

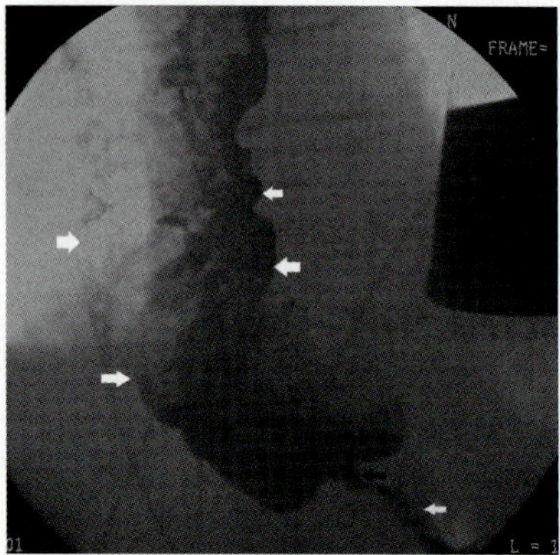

Figure 50.

Management

This patient has Chagas disease. He has developed complications that include megaesophagus and cardiomyopathy. Achalasia is defined as failure of relaxation of the lower esophageal sphincter, with loss of peristalsis of the distal esophagus. This occurs because of degeneration of the ganglion cells in the myenteric plexus in the esophageal wall. Patients with Chagas disease have an achalasia-like presentation, with dysphagia to solids and liquids, weight loss, and regurgitation of undigested food. Treatment is symptomatic as the disease process cannot be halted. The patient was probably infected by the protozoan when he traveled to South America years ago. He developed an early illness from which he recovered and is now experiencing the chronic phase of the disease.

With regard to treatment for his dysphagia, the patient should be referred to a gastroenterologist to discuss possible symptomatic treatment options. These include dilation of the lower esophageal sphincter, botulinum toxin injection, surgical myotomy, and calcium-channel blockers such as nifedipine for patients who are not surgical candidates.

The patient should be advised not to eat large meals while waiting for his GI appointment. He should also be referred for an echocardiogram in the next day or two. He should reduce his salt intake and follow-up with a cardiologist soon after obtaining the echocardiogram.

Clinical pearls

- Dysphagia to liquids is very uncommon, and is most often seen with achalasia and Chagas disease. Liquid dysphagia occurs only very late in esophageal or gastroesophageal junction carcinoma.
- Chagas disease presents with both an acute and chronic phase.
- Treatment is symptomatic, as the disease is progressive.
- Malignancy may also present with achalasia-like symptoms, and this should be ruled out with contrast radiography or endoscopy.

Impress your attending

What are the other complications of Chagas disease, other than cardiac and esophageal manifestations?

- Abscess formation.
- Adherence to the abdominal wall or other abdominal organs, which can lead to intestinal obstruction or intussusception.

Case 21

A 57-year-old man presents to the urgent clinic with abdominal pain. The pain began a few weeks ago but has become significantly worse in the past week. The patient says the pain is crampy in nature and located in the lower abdomen. It does not radiate, and the patient can identify no specific aggravating or relieving factors.

The patient also says he has been having frequent episodes of diarrhea, up to four times a day, for the past week. He passes mucus and has seen blood in the toilet bowl. He denies fever or weight loss. He feels slightly feverish. He is not experiencing joint symptoms. The patient is adopted and does not know anything about his biological parents. He has a mild degree of asthma and uses albuterol as needed. He is allergic to IV contrast, and had an anaphylactic reaction 5 years ago.

What is your differential diagnosis?

The differential diagnosis includes inflammatory bowel disease, colon cancer, infectious colitis, and irritable bowel syndrome.

Physical examination

Vitals Temperature 101.10F, HR 102 bpm, BP 110/70mmHg, oxygen saturation 99% on RA.

GEN No significant distress and does not appear unwell.

Hands Stage 3 clubbing.

H+N No scleral icterus or dry mucous membranes. No aphthous ulcers.

CVS Normal S1, S2. No murmurs, rubs, or gallops.

RESP C lear to auscultation.

ABD Diffusely tender but soft. No rigidity or guarding. Bowel sounds are present. Rectal examination reveals guaiac-positive stool.

EXT No edema.

What blood test(s) will you order?

CBC	WBC	15 x 10^3/μL with no left shift
	Hemoglobin	13.1g/dL
	Hematocrit	41.3%
	Platelets	324 x 10^3/μL
CHEM-7	Na	141mEq/L
	K	3.4mEq/L
	Cl	102mEq/L
	Bicarbonate	25mEq/L
	BUN	15mg/dL
	Creatinine	1.0mg/dL
	Glucose	95mg/dL
ESR		28mm/h
Lactate		1.0mmol/L

Stool culture and sensitivity are pending.

What do these laboratory data suggest?

The patient has an inflammatory or neoplastic process.

What is the ideal imaging test to help with your suspected diagnosis?

A CT scan of the abdomen and pelvis with oral and IV contrast. The images shown in Figures 51 and 52 are obtained.

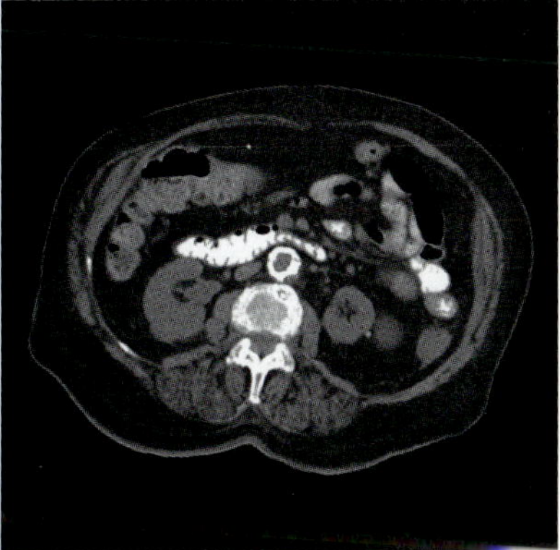

Figure 51.

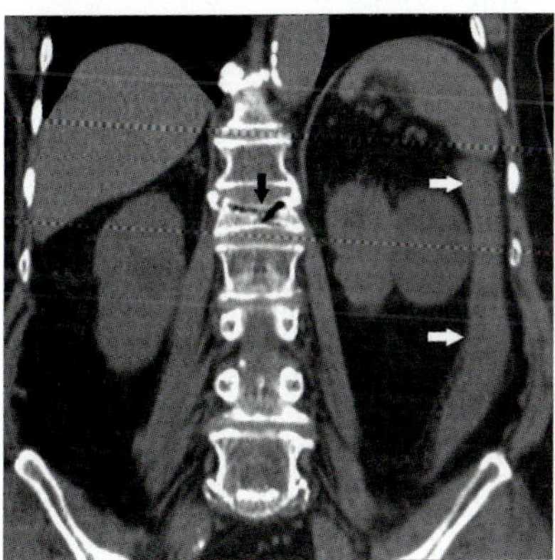

Figure 52.

Describe what you see and read on

These are axial (Figure 51) and coronal (Figure 52) views of the abdomen with oral contrast only; IV contrast was not given because of the history of anaphylaxis. There is marked colonic wall thickening of the descending colon, with a small amount of adjacent fluid and fat stranding. The normal haustral markings of the colon have been lost (white arrows). No adenopathy is seen. An upper lumbar vertebral compression fracture (black arrow) is incidentally noted, the age of which is indeterminate based on this scan.

The differential diagnosis for these findings includes an inflammatory cause such as ulcerative colitis or an infectious process. Although less likely, an ischemic etiology is also in the differential diagnosis.

What is the next step?

The patient should be treated for mild ulcerative colitis until a gastroenterology consultation can be arranged.

Assessing disease severity

Table 2 gives the criteria for disease severity in ulcerative colitis.

Given that this patient falls under the category of mild disease, and more importantly he does not look ill, he can be treated as an outpatient. Treatment for mild disease involves oral corticosteroids, sulfasalazine, or 5-aminosalicylic acid (oral or enemas). Sulfasalazine is a good choice as an initial daily option because it is effective, well tolerated, and not immune suppressing (should the patient turn out to have infectious or ischemic colitis after all). It should be continued until remission, which for most patients is about 3 weeks. A gastroenterologist will usually have seen the patient by this time. The gastroenterologist will confirm the suspected diagnosis and tailor therapy based on histopathology and the severity of the endoscopic appearance.

Table 2. Classifying disease severity in ulcerative colitis.

	Mild	Moderate	Severe
Bowel movements (no./day)	<4	4-6	>6
Temperature	Normal	Slightly elevated	Markedly elevated
Pulse (bpm)	<70	70-90	>90
Hemoglobin (g/dL)	>11	10.5-11	<10.5
ESR (mm/h)	<30	-	>30

This patient should have regular follow-up appointments with his primary-care physician and go to the emergency room if his symptoms worsen.

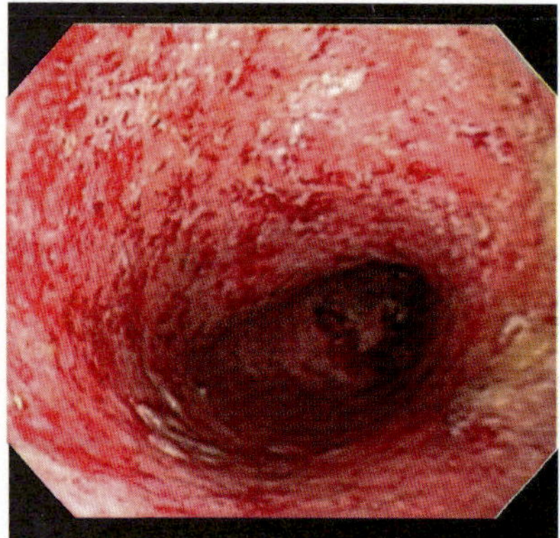

Figure 53.

Describe what you see and read on

The endoscopic picture of a similar patient shown in Figure 53 demonstrates the characteristic findings seen in ulcerative colitis, with erythema, edema, hemorrhage, and widespread scattered ulceration.

Clinical pearls

- Ulcerative colitis presents with crampy abdominal pain and diarrhea (often bloody), usually in the second or third decades of life. However, it can present later — as in this case.
- The disease is classified based on severity.
- Medications range from topical drugs for mild disease to oral agents, long-term steroids, and immunomodulators. A patient with an initial mild case of ulcerative colitis may not require maintenance therapy.
- Extraintestinal manifestations of ulcerative colitis include uveitis, episcleritis, erythema nodosum, pyoderma gangrenosum, large-joint arthritis, sclerosing cholangitis, and autoimmune hemolytic anemia.

Impress your attending

What are the key differences between ulcerative colitis and Crohn's disease?

- Ulcerative colitis affects the mucosal layer of the colon and rectum only, always involves the rectum, and spreads proximally in a continuous fashion.
- Crohn's disease is characterized by transmural inflammation and can present anywhere in the entire gut. Skip lesions will be seen.

What are the stages of clubbing?

Clubbing has many causes and is also an extraintestinal manifestation of ulcerative colitis. It has five stages:

- Stage 1: increased fluctuation of the nail bed.

- Stage 2: loss of angle between the nail and nail bed.
- Stage 3: increase in anteroposterior diameter.
- Stage 4: drumstick appearance.
- Stage 5: hypertrophic pulmonary osteoarthro-pathy.

Case 22

A 67-year-old man presents to the emergency room with diarrhea. He has been going to the bathroom at least 10 times a day for the past couple of days. The stools are mostly watery. He has cramps before each bowel movement, but no real pain. He has not seen blood on the paper or in the toilet. He has not traveled recently and has eaten the same foods as his family. No one else in his family is ill. He says his pants are fitting him better and thinks it is because he has lost some weight. He has no other past medical history. He has never had diarrhea like this before. A review of systems is negative for pulmonary or cardiac issues. However, the patient says his face and chest turn red and purple, which lasts up to a minute, whenever he eats or is involved in an emotional argument with his wife. He does not smoke or use illicit drugs.

Physical examination

Vitals Afebrile, HR 104 bpm, BP 100/55mmHg, oxygen saturation 99% on RA.

GEN No apparent distress.

HEENT No scleral icterus, but dry mucous membranes.

CVS Normal S1, S2. No murmurs, rubs, or gallops.

RESP Clear to auscultation.

ABD Soft and non-tender. No rigidity, guarding, or rebound tenderness. Liver span is 18cm. Bowel sounds are hyperactive. Rectal examination reveals an empty vault with no blood on the glove.

EXT No edema.

What is the most likely diagnosis?

The most likely diagnosis is a carcinoid tumor causing carcinoid syndrome. The differential diagnosis includes inflammatory bowel disease (especially ulcerative colitis), adenocarcinoma of the colon, microscopic colitis, and systemic mastocytosis.

What blood test(s) will you order?

CBC	WBC	10.7 x 10^3/μL
	Hemoglobin	14.7g/dL
	Hematocrit	38.8%
	Platelets	207 x 10^3/μL
CHEM-7	Na	142mEq/L
	K	4.3mEq/L
	Cl	102mEq/L
	Bicarbonate	25mEq/L
	BUN	27mg/dL
	Creatinine	1.1mg/dL
	Glucose	99mg/dL

What do these laboratory data suggest?

Given the BUN to creatinine ratio is more than 20:1, the renal laboratory data point toward a possible prerenal cause of kidney injury.

Given the most likely diagnosis, what urine test should be ordered?

A 24-hour urine looking for elevated levels of 5-hydroxyindoleacetic acid is the diagnostic test of choice. Serotonin levels can also be checked for elevation.

What imaging test will you order?

A CT scan of the abdomen and pelvis is obtained (Figures 54 and 55).

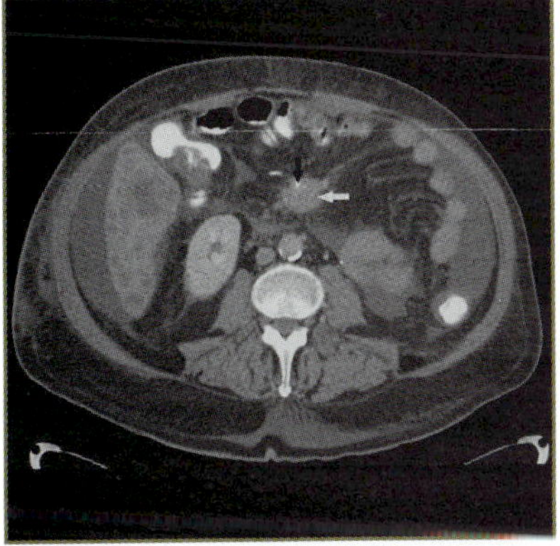

Figure 54.

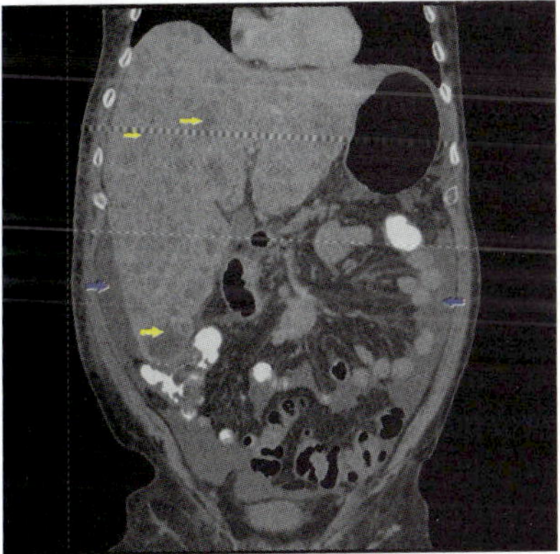

Figure 55.

Describe what you see and read on

Axial (Figure 54) and coronal (Figure 55) images with IV and oral contrast are obtained. There is a soft-tissue mass (white arrow) measuring up to 3cm in the midline anterior to the aorta and left renal vein. The mass is not adherent to any loops of bowel and is located in the mesentery. It encases the superior mesenteric artery (black arrow) but is not compressing it. The liver is enlarged and demonstrates numerous hypodensities (yellow arrows) of various sizes, some of which are soft-tissue density. Ascites is seen in both paracolic gutters (blue arrows), around the liver, and in the pelvis. The visualized loops of small bowel and colon are normal in size.

Given the soft-tissue mass with numerous lesions in the liver, metastatic disease is the most likely diagnosis. Together with the patient's symptoms, these findings are consistent with a metastatic carcinoid tumor causing carcinoid syndrome.

What other imaging modalities can be used to make this diagnosis?

- MRI — this is a very sensitive imaging modality for identifying hepatic metastases, especially during the hepatic-arterial phase (hypervascular metastases) and on T2-weighted sequences.
- Octreotide scan — many carcinoid tumors have somatostatin receptors. Administering a somatostatin analog such as octreotide and imaging the entire body will allow localization of the tumor.

What is the next step?

The patient has metastatic disease, and therefore the goal is to control symptoms. Carcinoid syndrome is caused by the tumor synthesizing and releasing various polypeptides, biogenic amines, and prostaglandins, which are inactivated by the liver. With decreasing liver mass because of metastases to the liver, and increasing production of these bioactive agents by the expanding tumor burden, the residual liver becomes unable to cope with the overwhelming amount of these substances. The result is the symptom complex characteristic of carcinoid syndrome.

This patient needs to be admitted to the medical ward for rehydration to correct his renal injury. The long-term goals of treatment will be supportive, including avoiding situations that induce flushing episodes, cessation of alcohol ingestion, and avoiding trauma to the right upper quadrant. Octreotide can be administered subcutaneously and titrated to the optimum dose needed for symptom relief. In patients refractory to octreotide, serotonin antagonists or interferon therapy can be used.

Surgical resection is an option for patients who present with a solitary tumor, with or without an isolated metastasis.

Clinical pearls

- Carcinoid syndrome is a constellation of symptoms that encompass flushing, diarrhea, bronchospasm, and dyspnea/heart failure symptoms.
- The patient's history can be classic for the diagnosis.
- Urinary 5-hydroxyindoleacetic acid and serotonin levels can aid in diagnosis.
- CT, MRI, and octreotide scans are the imaging modalities of choice.
- Supportive measures, along with octreotide, are first-line therapy for reducing symptoms.

Impress your attending

At what locations in the body do carcinoid tumors typically present?

Appendix, small intestine, rectum, stomach, colon, and bronchi.

Carcinoid tumors affect the heart. What is the pathophysiology and what symptoms do patients have?

Plaque-like deposits form on the cusps of valves. This most commonly (90% of cases) occurs on the right side of the heart and more specifically at the tricuspid valve. Patients present initially with fatigue and dyspnea on exertion, followed by more overt signs and symptoms of right heart failure.

Case 23

A 67-year-old man presents to the hospital with abdominal pain. The pain is located in the epigastric region and is best described as a gnawing pain that does not radiate. It began a week ago and arises intermittently. His symptoms have been getting progressively worse, and he decided to seek medical attention today after having two episodes of coffee-ground emesis in the past 24 hours. He rates the abdominal pain as 8/10 in severity. The pain is aggravated by eating.

Associated symptoms include feeling lightheaded or dizzy at times. The patient's bowel habits are unchanged and he has not had black stools. He does not experience symptoms of gastroesophageal reflux disease. His past medical history includes osteoarthritis of the knees, gout, and asthma, which are all relatively well controlled. He does not smoke or drink alcohol. Medications include albuterol as needed and ibuprofen 600mg three times a day. He was discharged from the hospital 10 days ago after a flare-up of his asthma. The remainder of the systems review is non-contributory.

Physical examination

Vitals Afebrile, HR 110 bpm, BP 105/55mmHg, oxygen saturation 97% on RA.

GEN A well-built, muscular man.

Hands No clubbing. Normal-appearing palmar creases.

HEENT No jaundice or lymphadenopathy. Dry mucous membranes.

CVS Normal S1, S2. No murmurs, rubs, or gallops.

RESP Clear to auscultation.

ABD Tenderness in the epigastric region. No rigidity, guarding, or rebound tenderness. Bowel sounds are normal. Rectal examination reveals brown stool (stool occult-negative).

EXT No edema.

What additional vital sign will you obtain?

Orthostatic blood pressure:

Supine	105/60mmHg
Sitting	100/55mmHg
Standing	90/50mmHg

What diagnosis does the history and physical examination suggest?

The history suggests a diagnosis of an upper GI bleed secondary to peptic ulcer disease.

What blood test(s) will you order?

CBC	WBC	8.9 x 10³/μL
	Hemoglobin	12.5g/dL
	Hematocrit	35.7%
	Platelets	330 x 10³/μL
CHEM-7	Na	140mEq/L

	K	3.6mEq/L
	Cl	100mEq/L
	Bicarbonate	25mEq/L
	BUN	45mg/dL
	Creatinine	0.9mg/dL
	Glucose	89mg/dL
INR		1.0

These laboratory data suggest mild anemia. The elevated BUN level is a result of absorption of blood by the small intestine, as well as dehydration.

The patient calls to you from behind the curtain — he has just vomited frank red blood.

How will you manage this patient in the immediate setting?

The main focus is to make sure the patient is maintaining his airway. If this were an obtunded individual, intubation to protect the airway from aspiration would be the next step. However, this patient is awake and alert and has no issues with respiration.

The next step is to assess the circulation. The patient's vital signs during the examination show he is already tachycardic and orthostatic. Two large-bore IV lines should be placed, starting aggressive hydration with an isotonic solution (normal saline or lactated Ringer's). Additional blood work including a type and screen should be requested. A gastroenterology consultation should be obtained for an urgent upper endoscopy, and a nasogastric tube should be placed and maintained on continuous suction. The patient should be started on a high-dose IV proton-pump inhibitor.

What is the value of the nasogastric tube?

The nasogastric tube is placed, and saline is instilled into the stomach and then withdrawn. Withdrawal of bloody fluid will indicate ongoing bleeding, while dark coffee-ground material will indicate clotted or old blood. A negative lavage can either mean the bleeding has stopped or the tip of the nasogastric tube did not reach the site of bleeding.

In this patient, only clotted blood and coffee grounds are seen in the suction trap. The gastroenterologist decides the patient is stable enough to delay EGD until later in the day.

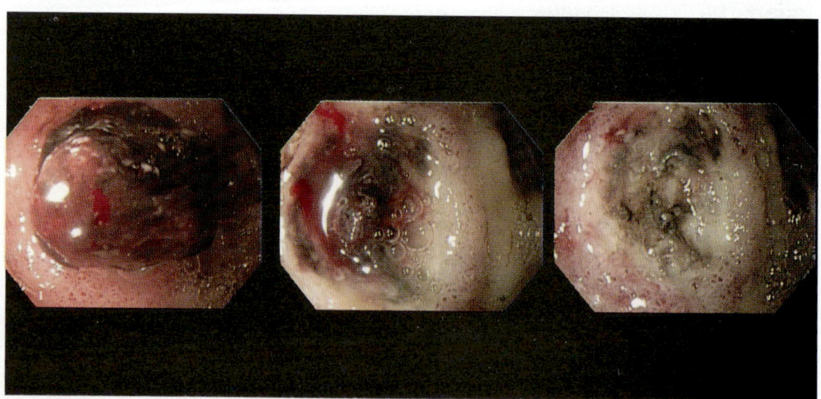

Figure 56.

Imaging

The EGD is performed and the images shown in Figure 56 are obtained.

Describe what you see and read on

suggestive of recent bleeding. The second photo shows the ulcer after injection of a 1:10,000

The first endoscopic photo shows a 12mm duodenal ulcer crater with an adherent clot dilutionof epinephrine in saline (note blanching of the mucosa); the clot has been removed with a snare. An artery is present, with an overlying brown clot in the base of the ulcer. Despite an epinephrine injection, blood is still oozing from the artery. The third photo shows the appearance after cauterization of the artery with a bipolar electrocautery probe.

How will you manage this patient after the EGD?

Given there has been no further bleeding, the patient's volume status should be assessed (remember, he was hypotensive when he initially presented). The ulcer should be treated with a twice-daily oral proton-pump inhibitor for 5 days, followed by standard-dose therapy for 8 weeks. The patient has been taking ibuprofen, which is a risk factor for the development of duodenal ulcers, but it would be wise to check a serum antibody or stool antigen for *Helicobacter pylori* if biopsies of the antrum were not taken during the EGD.

This patient has had arthritis for years and has been on the same dose of ibuprofen.

Why would he suddenly develop ulcers now?

This patient was recently discharged from the hospital for an asthma exacerbation, which probably included a daily dose of steroids. The risk of bleeding increases significantly when steroids are combined with NSAIDs.

Clinical pearl

- Taking steroids with NSAIDs greatly increases the risk of a peptic ulcer and peptic ulcer bleeding.

Impress your attending

What are some other causes of upper GI bleeding?

- Esophageal or gastric varices.
- AV malforma tions.
- Mallory-Weiss tear.
- Erosions.
- Benign tumors (leiomyoma).
- Malignancy (adenocarcinoma, squamous cell carcinoma, GI stromal tumor, lymphoma).
- Dieulafoy lesion.
- Iatrogenic (following sphincterotomy or percutaneous endoscopic gastrostomy).

Case 24

A 35-year-old woman with no significant past medical history presents to the emergency room with diffuse abdominal pain 2 weeks after a difficult laparoscopic cholecystectomy. The patient was discharged a day after the cholecystectomy with minimal postoperative pain, but presented to the clinic a few days later with bloating and crampy abdominal discomfort. The surgeon's impression was constipation, and he prescribed a laxative. Since then, she says, her pain has increased.

The patient describes her pain as a dull tightness mostly in the right upper quadrant, but radiating to her back and right shoulder. The pain is constant and she rates it as 7/10 in intensity. There are no specific aggravating or relieving factors. Associated symptoms include abdominal distension and nausea. She denies fever, chills, or sweats. The patient's family history and social history are non-contributory. Current medications include docusate sodium for constipation and acetaminophen with codeine for pain control.

Physical examination

Vitals Afebrile, HR 90 bpm, BP 120/75mmHg, oxygen saturation 98% on RA.

GEN Appears to be in moderate distress.

Hands No clubbing or muscle wasting.

H+N Positive for scleral icterus. No adenopathy. No fetor hepaticus.

CVS Normal S1, S2. No murmurs, rubs, or gallops.

RESP Decreased breath sounds at the right base. No egophony.

ABD Abdomen appears distended. No tenderness. No rigidity, guarding, or rebound tenderness. Dullness to percussion is noted throughout. Shifting dullness is positive. Bowel sounds are hypoactive. Rectal examination reveals an empty vault.

EXT No edema.

What is the most likely diagnosis?

Given the patient has postoperative jaundice and fluid in the abdomen, and has undergone recent surgery, a bile leak is the most likely diagnosis.

What blood test(s) will you order?

CBC	WBC	14.9 x $10^3/\mu L$
	Hemoglobin	13.5g/dL
	Hematocrit	38.8%
	Platelets	553 x$10^3/\mu L$
CHEM-7	Na	139mEq/L
	K	3.8mEq/L
	Cl	104mEq/L
	Bicarbonate	23mEq/L

	BUN	11mg/dL
	Creatinine	0.6mg/dL
	Glucose	112mg/dL
LFTs	AST	53 units/L
	ALT	64 units/L
	Alkaline phosphatase	110 units/L
	Total bilirubin	2.9mg/dL

Imaging

A CT scan of the abdomen and pelvis is obtained by the emergency-room physician (Figure 57).

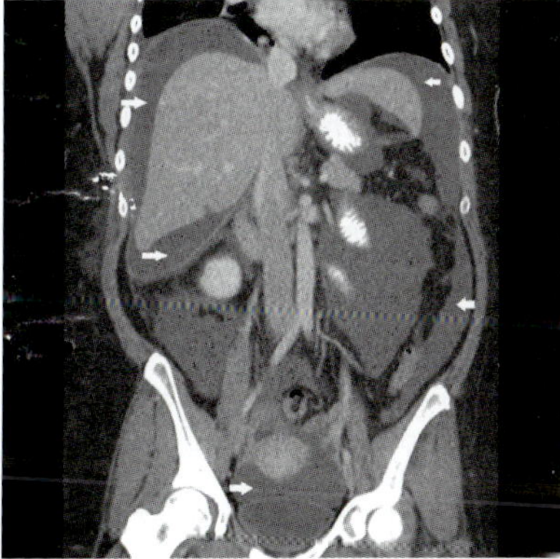

Figure 57.

Describe what you see and read on

A single coronal CT image with IV and oral contrast is shown. There is a large amount of free intraperitoneal fluid (white arrows) in the perihepatic, subhepatic, and perisplenic regions. Fluid is also noted in the left paracolic gutter, as well as within the pelvis. The visualized portions of the liver are smooth and normal in size. Given these findings and the recent cholecystectomy, a bile leak remains the most likely etiology. The patient should have a therapeutic paracentesis at this point to help alleviate the discomfort. A percutaneous drain can be left in place if definitive therapy cannot be arranged within 24 hours.

How will you confirm a bile leak?

You can do either a HIDA scan or obtain a gastroenterology consultation for an ERCP An image from a HIDA scan demonstrating a bile leak is shown (Figure 58).

HIDA scans are performed by injecting about 10mCi of IV Tc99m disofenin and obtaining dynamic imaging of the upper abdomen in the anterior view for around 30 minutes. Activity is typically initially noted in the liver, followed by the gallbladder and common bile duct.

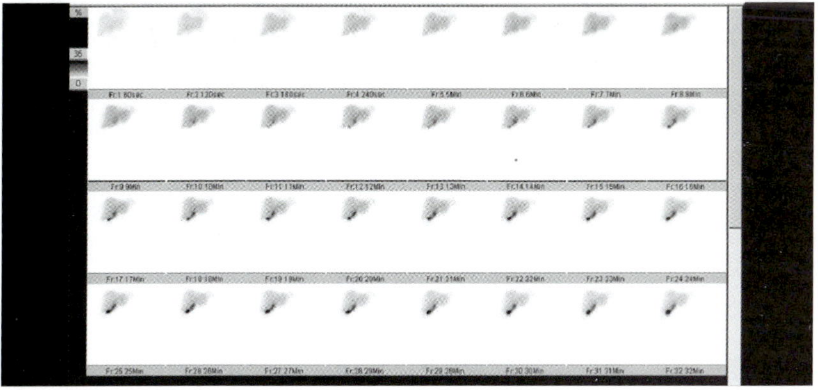

Figure 58.

Small-bowel activity confirms the biliary tract is connected. On the examination shown above, foci of extraluminal activity are identified in the gallbladder fossa, around the liver, and in the right paracolic gutter. No activity is seen in the distal common bile duct or small bowel. This suggests a high probability that the common bile duct is transected. If this was a blow out of the cystic duct, then a little activity in the common bile duct and small bowel would have been seen on the HIDA scan.

An ERCP is then obtained (Figure 59).

Describe what you see and read on

This single fluoroscopic image over the right upper quadrant during ERCP demonstrates contrast was injected into the distal common bile duct (white arrow). The pancreatic duct is barely visible just to the right of L1 (black arrow). The common bile duct courses for a length of about 4cm, as measured from the ampulla, and shows a normal caliber. There is immediate contrast extravasation, presumably from the junction of the common hepatic duct and the common duct, with contrast collecting in the subhepatic region (yellow arrow). This indicates an injury of the biliary duct system in the area of the upper aspect of the common bile duct.

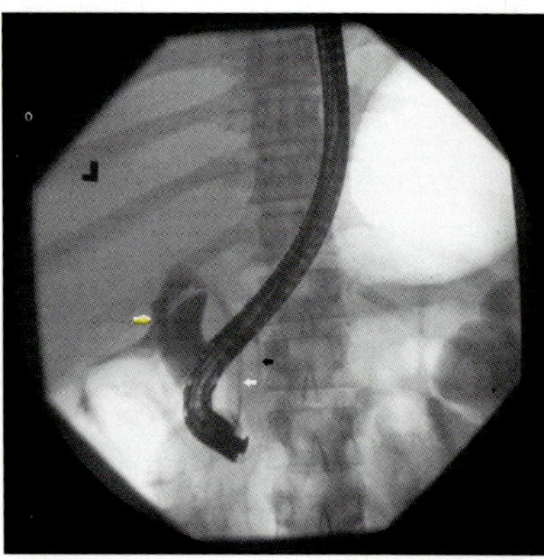

Figure 59.

Now that a biliary leak is confirmed, what is the next step in management?

Repair of the leak is the next step. This can be done either surgically or endoscopically with a biliary stent.

A repeat retrograde cholangiogram is attempted (Figure 60).

Describe what you see and read on

The initial image on the left shows contrast injection into the common bile

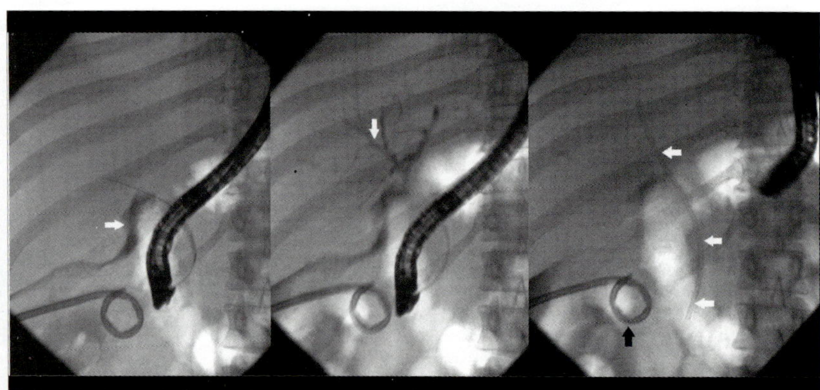

Figure 60.

duct with rapid extravasation (white arrow) from the proximal aspect of the common hepatic duct. The middle image shows cannulation into the hepatic ducts without complete filling of the intrahepatic bile ducts (white arrow). The cystic duct is not filled. The final image on the right shows a biliary stent advanced into the intrahepatic ducts, clearly bridging the leak with its distal aspect within the duodenal lumen (white arrows). A percutaneous drain is also noted (black arrow).

Once the patient returns to the ward, she should remain nil by mouth except for oral medications. Her diet can be advanced the next day if there are no signs of complications such as pancreatitis. Anticoagulants should be held for approximately 10 days.

This patient has an indwelling percutaneous pigtail drain, as shown above. When drain output of bile ceases, the leak is presumed to have healed. Repeat ERCP should then be performed to retrieve the stent and confirm resolution of the bile leak. Complete transections of the common bile duct are an extremely uncommon complication of biliary tract surgery, and biliary continuity can only rarely be re-established with ERCP alone. When stented, the bile duct usually heals with a stricture (this is ischemic in origin), and long-term stenting or hepaticojejunostomy is usually needed.

Clinical pearls

- A patient presenting with jaundice and abdominal distension after cholecystectomy is most likely experiencing a bile leak.
- Biliary injury is classified as follows by Strasberg *et al*[1]:

  - Type A: leak from a minor duct still in continuity with the common bile duct;

  - Type B: occlusion of part of the biliary tree; - Type C: bile leak from a duct not in communication with the common bile duct;

  - Type D: lateral injury to the extrahepatic bile

    duct;

  - Type E: circumferential injury to a major bile duct.

Impress your attending

What are the ducts of Luschka?

These are small, intrahepatic bile ducts adjacent to the gallbladder fossa, originating from the right hepatic lobe. They are sometimes injured when the gallbladder is dissected from the liver bed, resulting in a bile leak from the intrahepatic, right-sided bile ducts.

Reference

1. Strasberg SM, Hertl M, Soper NJ. An analysis of the problem of biliary injury during laparoscopic cholecystectomy. *J Am Coll Surg* 1995; 180: 101-25.

Case 25

A 40-year-old woman presents to the emergency department with abdominal pain. The pain is located in the right upper quadrant. It began about 30 minutes after the patient ate a fried chicken meal. She describes the pain as crampy in nature, radiating to the epigastric region. She rates it as 7/10 in severity. The patient took Percocet at home, but this did not relieve the pain.

Associated symptoms include fever and nausea. The patient presented to her primary-care physician a few weeks ago with vague abdominal pain that subsided. The work-up revealed cholelithiasis, for which she postponed a cholecystectomy until after the coming holidays.

What is your differential diagnosis?

The differential diagnosis includes cholangitis, choledocholithiasis, and cholecystitis.

Physical examination

Vitals Temperature 102.3°F, HR 120 bpm, BP 115/65mmHg, oxygen saturation 97% on RA.

GEN An overweight woman who appears to be in distress.

Hands No clubbing. Normal-appearing palmar creases.

HEENT Scleral icterus and dry mucous membranes. No lymphadenopathy.

CVS Normal S1, S2. No murmurs, rubs, or gallops.

RESP Clear to auscultation.

ABD Tenderness in the right upper quadrant. No rigidity, guarding, or rebound tenderness. Murphy's sign is negative. Bowel sounds are normal. Rectal examination reveals brown stool (occult-negative).

EXT No edema.

Skin Mild jaundice.

What blood test(s) will you order?

CBC	WBC	14.9 x $10^3/\mu L$
	Hemoglobin	12.7g/dL
	Hematocrit	38.7%
	Platelets	320 x $10^3/\mu L$
CHEM-7	Na	140mEq/L
	K	3.9mEq/L
	Cl	103mEq/L
	Bicarbonate	23mEq/L
	BUN	12mg/dL
	Creatinine	1.0mg/dL
	Glucose	89mg/dL
LFTs	AST	160 units/L
	ALT	730 units/L
	Alkaline phosphatase	253 units/L
	Total bilirubin	5.4mg/dL

Lipase	26 units/L
INR	1.0

These laboratory data suggest an infectious process is occurring, as well as an obstructive process based on the liver-associated enzymes. The bilirubin level is also elevated, which correlates with the physical examination findings of jaundice and scleral icterus.

What imaging test will you order first?

The first imaging study should be an ultrasound of the right upper quadrant. This again confirms the presence of gallstones, but there is no sonographic evidence of cholecystitis. The common bile duct is dilated up to 1cm, and the intrahepatic ducts are also dilated. Choledocholithiasis is not seen.

What is the next step?

The next step is to seek a GI consultation for a possible ERCP. This is because ultrasound does not always detect stones in the common bile duct. Although fever and right upper quadrant pain can be seen with acute cholecystitis, the absence of gallbladder wall thickening, pericholecystic fluid, and sonographic Murphy's sign suggest that acute cholecystitis is not present. These symptoms (fever, right upper quadrant pain, and jaundice) and the dilated intra- and extrahepatic bile ducts suggest the patient has an occluded common bile duct resulting in cholangitis. The patient should be kept nil by mouth, placed on IV fluids, started on a broad-spectrum antibiotic such as ampicillin-sulbactam, piperacillin-tazobactam, or a fluoroquinolone, and sent to the regular medical/surgical ward.

The patient undergoes ERCP the next day (Figure 61).

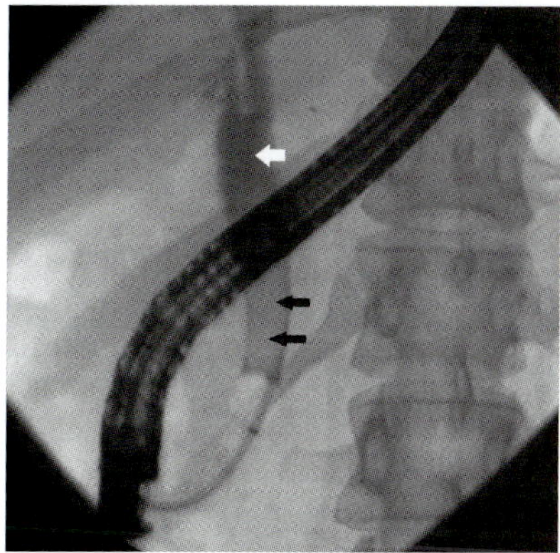

Figure 61.

Describe what you see and read on

A single image during the retrograde cholangiogram demonstrates an endoscope in place, with a guidewire in the common bile and hepatic ducts. The gastroenterologist's report says a sphincterotomy was performed and a large yellow stone passed through the duct.

The common bile duct is opacified with contrast and measures up to 11mm (white arrow). A smooth sausage-shaped filling defect is present in the common bile duct proximal to the balloon (black arrows). This is a large air bubble resulting from reflux of air after biliary sphincterotomy.

The patient's symptoms are greatly improved after the procedure. The post-procedure plan includes monitoring on the ward, continuing antibiotics, and advancing her diet as tolerated. Her LFTs should also be monitored to document they are trending downward. By the time of discharge the patient is pain-free and tolerating a diet, and her enzymes have markedly decreased.

Discharge data

LFTs	AST	80 units/L
	ALT	300 units/L
	Alkaline phosphatase	70 units/L
	Total bilirubin	2.1mg/dL

She is advised to follow-up with her surgeon after the holidays.

The patient presents back to the hospital a week later with similar symptoms to the initial hospitalization. She does not appear as jaundiced this time, but the physical examination is notable for a positive Murphy's sign. Initial laboratory data show an alkaline phosphatase level of 300 units/L and an ALT level of 450 units/L. Bedside ultrasound shows gallbladder wall thickening, pericholecystic fluid, and shadowing gallstones. The common bile duct is now normal in size, but the intrahepatic ducts are still dilated. A diagnosis of acute cholecystitis is made, and the patient is started on antibiotics and taken to the operating room.

During the cholecystectomy, an intraoperative cholangiogram is performed (Figure 62).

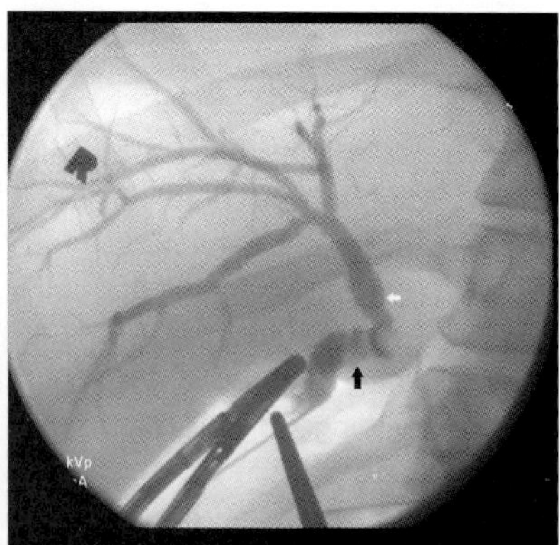

Figure 62. *Image Coutesy of Dr. Peter Ghobrial.*

Describe what you see and read on

Contrast is injected into the distal cystic duct. The image shows a large obstructing filling defect in the most proximal cystic duct (black arrow), apparently medially and anteriorly. This is compressing the common hepatic duct, causing moderate dilatation of the common hepatic duct (white arrow) and central bile ducts. This is consistent with a diagnosis of Mirizzi syndrome.

This patient initially presented with an obstructing stone in the common bile duct, and the stone was removed. However, she had cholelithiasis and was at risk of more stones passing into the cystic duct or common bile duct. In this case, a stone or stones impacted in the cystic duct caused obstruction of the common hepatic duct, a phenomenon known as Mirizzi syndrome. Mirizzi syndrome can also result from extrinsic compression caused by an impacted stone in Hartmann's pouch of the gallbladder.

This patient should receive standard post-cholecystectomy care and can be discharged as soon as her postoperative pain is controlled and she is tolerating a diet. She should follow-up with her surgeon in 1-2 weeks.

Clinical pearls

- Mirizzi syndrome refers to obstruction of the common hepatic duct caused by an extrinsic compression from an impacted stone in the cystic duct or Hartmann's pouch.
- Surgery is the main treatment for Mirizzi syndrome, if the diagnosis is made preoperatively.
- Temporizing measures prior to surgery include endoscopic stent

placement to relieve the obstruction until definitive surgical therapy can be offered.

Impress your attending

What is the original classification by McSherry of Mirizzi syndrome? [1]

- Type 1: compression of the common hepatic duct or common bile duct by a stone in the cystic duct or Hartmann's pouch.
- Type 2: erosion of the calculus from the cystic duct into the common hepatic duct or common bile duct, therefore causing a cholecystocholedochal fistula that is less than 1800 of the circumference of the common bile duct. (If ≤180°, the defect can be repaired surgically over a T-tube.)
- Type 3: as for type 2, but with more than 180° of injury. This cannot be repaired over a T-tube; hepaticojejunostomy is required.
- Type 4: complete transection or obliteration of the common bile duct by pressure necrosis or inflammation from the compressing stone. This also requires hepaticojejunostomy.

Reference

1. McSherry CK, Ferstenberg H, Virshup M. The Mirizzi syndrome: suggested classification and surgical treatment. *Surg Gastroenterol* 1982; 1: 219.

Case 26

A 65-year-old woman arrives at the emergency room after two episodes of vomiting bright-red blood. The patient has no abdominal pain or history of nausea. The latest vomiting episode did not follow a meal, and occurred a few hours before presentation to the emergency room. Her bowel motions have been normal so far, and she denies bright-red blood per rectum or melena. She has experienced no fevers, chills, or weight loss.

The patient is known to have autoimmune hepatitis that was diagnosed 8 months ago. This was found as part of investigations for abnormal LFTs and she underwent a liver biopsy at the time. Her other past medical history is significant for hypothyroidism, dyslipidemia, and hypertension. Her home medications include simvastatin, levothyroxine, prednisone, and azathioprine. She drinks alcohol only occasionally and does not smoke. Her family history includes rheumatoid arthritis, but is unremarkable for GI disease. In the emergency room, she is found to be slightly tachycardic but with stable vital signs otherwise. Large-bore IV access is established and basic laboratory tests are requested. A nasogastric tube is placed and reveals bright-red blood. Irrigation with normal saline fails to clear the bloody contents.

What is your differential diagnosis?

The differential diagnosis includes peptic ulcer bleeding, gastritis, esophageal variceal bleeding, and a Mallory-Weiss tear.

Physical examination

Vitals Temperature 98.5°F, HR 110 bpm, BP 136/80mmHg, oxygen saturation 98% on RA.

GEN No obvious distress.

HEENT Moist mucous membranes. No scleral icterus. No lymphadenopathy.

CVS Normal S1, S2. No murmurs, rubs, or gallops.

RESP Clear to auscultation.

ABD Soft and non-tender. No appreciable ascites or palpable splenomegaly. Rectal examination reveals guaiac-negative stool.

EXT No clubbing or edema.

What blood test(s) will you order?

CBC	WBC	11 x 10^3/μL
	Hemoglobin	8.5g/dL
	Hematocrit	24%
	Platelets	56 x 10^3/μL
CHEM-7	Na	128mEq/L
	K	4.3mEq/L
	Cl	113mEq/L
	Bicarbonate	20mEq/L
	BUN	36mg/dL
	Creatinine	0.8mg/dL
	Glucose	130mg/dL

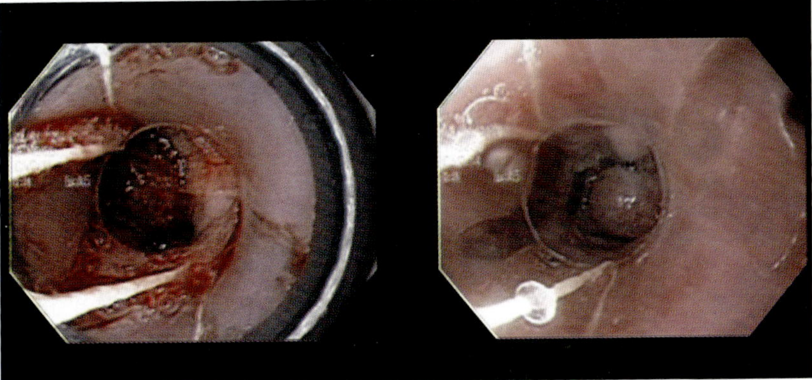

Figure 63.

	LFTs	AST
	ALT	74 units/L
	Alkaline phosphatase 130 units/L	
	Total bilirubin	1.2mg/dL
INR		1.1

Does this narrow your differential diagnosis?

Yes, it does. Clinically the patient is hemodynamically unstable, with tachycardia as well as evidence of positive bloody output through the nasogastric tube. The known diagnosis of autoimmune hepatitis with the presence of thrombocytopenia raises concern for cirrhosis and portal hypertension, and therefore possible esophageal variceal bleeding.

How will you proceed?

The next step is to obtain an emergent upper endoscopy. Prior to endoscopy, the patient should be started on IV octreotide to decrease her portal pressure. Parenteral antibiotics such as ceftriaxone or ciprofloxacin for Gram-negative bacteria should be started to prevent sepsis in the setting of possible bacterial translocation. An EGD is performed (Figure 63).

Describe what you see and read on

The EGD reveals a large grade 3 varix with stigmata of active bleeding. The varix is banded (image on right) with evidence of subsequent hemostasis.

With endoscopic variceal banding for primary hemorrhage control completed, octreotide should be continued for approximately 72 hours after endoscopy, and non-selective beta-blocker treatment should begin.

The patient undergoes a CT scan for other indications (Figure 64).

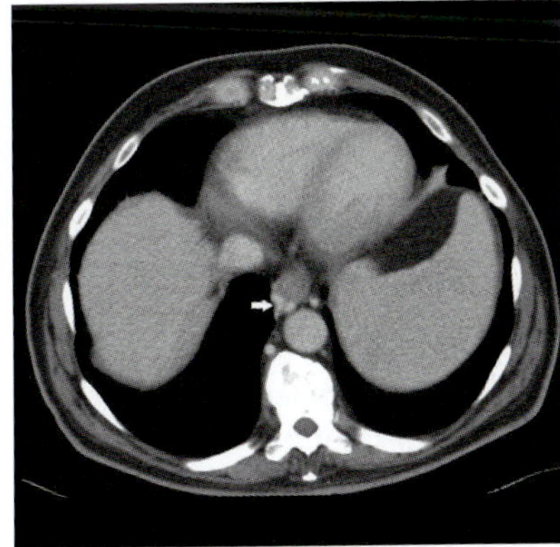

Figure 64. *Image Coutesy of Dr. Njogu Njuguna.*

Describe what you see and read on

This contrast-enhanced CT axial image through the upper abdomen shows prominent esophageal varices (white arrow) as well as splenomegaly.

Clinical pearls

- Esophageal variceal bleeding should be suspected in any patient with risk factors for cirrhosis who presents with GI bleeding.
- Thrombocytopenia is an especially important clue that a patient has cirrhosis, and should always prompt a working diagnosis of cirrhosis when seen in a patient with known or suspected liver disease. Other indications that a patient may be cirrhotic include a history of liver disease, laboratory findings (elevated INR, bilirubin, AST/ALT, and hypoalbuminemia), and clinical findings (cutaneous stigmata of cirrhosis, hepatosplenomegaly, and ascites).
- Refractory bleeding, or bleeding despite endoscopic band ligation, requires coil embolization. A transjugular intrahepatic portosystemic shunt is used for long-term management. This procedure creates an artificial shunt through a branch of the portal vein to a branch of the hepatic vein, resulting in decreased portal pressure.

Impress your attending

How would you predict mortality after atransjugular intrahepatic portosystemic shunt?

The MELD (Model for End-Stage Liver Disease) score is used. This is based on the INR, creatinine, and total bilirubin. It is also used to determine status on liver transplant waiting lists.

What are some contraindications to this procedure?

Pulmonary hypertension, complete portal vein thrombosis, severe end-stage liver disease (Child-Pugh class C, high MELD score), right heart failure, certain types of valvular heart disease, and refractory hepatic encephalopathy.

What are some complications?

Worsening liver failure may occur because of shunting of portal blood (the majority of the hepatic blood supply). Hepatic encephalopathy can also occur after shunt creation, particularly in older patients. Stenosis on either side of the shunt as well as occlusion are other complications.

Case 27

A 45-year-old woman is brought to the hospital by her husband, who has noticed a yellowing of her eyes and skin over the past 4 days. The patient is a busy lawyer and rarely seeks medical attention. She describes some right upper quadrant abdominal pain, which is mild and non-radiating. In addition, she has experienced nausea and anorexia over the past few days. She denies vomiting, diarrhea, constipation, melena, hematochezia, or pale-colored stools.

Her past medical and surgical history is unremarkable, apart from a hysterectomy for fibroids several years ago. She has two children and lives with her husband. She is a previous smoker, having quit 15 years ago. She drinks at least three glasses of wine each day with dinner. She does admit to drinking more at times, particularly on weekends and at business meetings. She has not traveled recently outside of the continental US, and has never received a blood transfusion or used IV drugs. She denies using cocaine or other illicit drugs. She is not taking prescription medications, over-the-counter substances, or herbal remedies. There is no family history of liver disease and no jaundice or GI symptoms have been reported in the past.

What is your differential diagnosis?

The differential diagnosis includes acute viral hepatitis, drug-induced liver injury/toxic hepatitis, alcoholic hepatitis, chronic alcoholic liver disease/cirrhosis, cholecystitis, choledocholithiasis, primary biliary cirrhosis, and primary sclerosing cholangitis.

Physical examination

Vitals Temperature 98.5°F, HR 90 bpm, BP 130/70mmHg, oxygen saturation 99% on RA.

GEN No obvious distress.

Hands No clubbing.

HEENT Icterus and dry mucous membranes. No lymphadenopathy.

CVS Normal S1, S2. No murmurs, rubs, or gallops.

RESP Clear to auscultation.

ABD Mild right upper quadrant tenderness causing pain on palpation. No rebound tenderness. No guarding. Two-fingerbreadth hepatomegaly. No splenomegaly appreciated. Bowel sounds are normal.

Skin No palmar erythema or spider angiomas.

NEURO Alert and oriented to time, place, and person. No asterixis.

What blood test(s) will you order?

CBC	WBC	18.0 x 10^3/µL
	Hemoglobin	9.0g/dL
	Hematocrit	29%

	Platelets	50 x 10^3/µL
	MCV	105fL/cell
CHEM-7	**Na**	133mEq/L
	K	4.4mEq/L
	Cl	110mEq/L
	Bicarbonate	22mEq/L
	BUN	21mg/dL
	Creatinine	0.9mg/dL
	Glucose	98mg/dL
LFTs	**AST**	280 units/L
	ALT	90 units/L
	Alkaline phosphatase	210 units/L
	Total bilirubin	13.3mg/dL (direct 10.0mg/dL)
	GGT	255 units/L
INR		2.2

Does this change your differential diagnosis?

The patient's examination reveals mildly tender hepatomegaly without cutaneous or other signs of chronic liver disease. Her LFTs are elevated, and her AST to ALT ratio is more than 2:1. In addition, her total bilirubin and GGT levels are markedly elevated. Her platelet count is low. Furthermore, the patient's social history suggests excessive alcohol intake. Other causes of an obstructive pattern of liver disease (such as gallstone disease) are possible and should be ruled out with an ultrasound. Given the patient's picture of acute hepatitis, acute viral hepatitis should also be ruled out. Primary biliary cirrhosis usually has a chronic history and is associated with severe pruritus.

Additional laboratory tests

Hepatitis C antibody	Negative
Hepatitis C RNA (quantification)	Negative
Hepatitis B surface antigen	Negative
Hepatitis B surface antibody	Negative
Hepatitis B core IgM antibody	Negative
Acetaminophen level	Undetectable
ANA	1:20
Anti-smooth muscle antibody	1:20
Serum IgG	1200mg/dL

What imaging test will you order?

The next step is to obtain an ultrasound of the right upper quadrant (Figure 65).

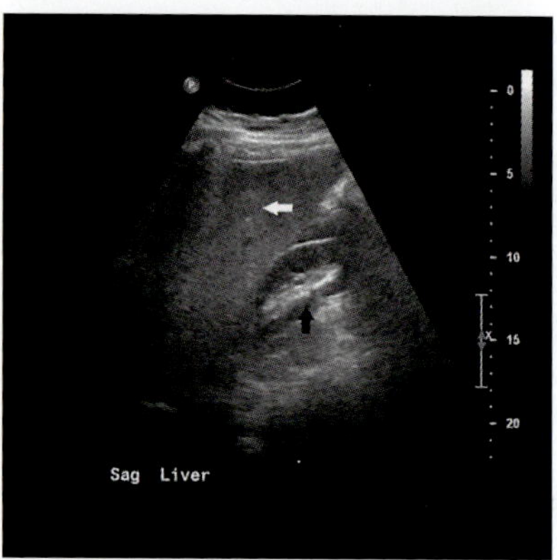

Figure 65.

Describe what you see and read on

A sagittal view of the liver demonstrates an echogenic liver (white arrow) as compared with the right kidney (black arrow). No focal hepatic lesions are identified. Although not shown on this image, the liver is noted to be shrunken. Ascites is not seen. The findings are consistent with hepatocellular disease.

How will you manage this patient?

The ultrasound has ruled out a focal lesion, but has raised the possibility of longstanding liver disease. In addition, other etiologies of the patient's acute hepatitis with an obstructive pattern have been ruled out. The next step is to return to the patient's family. They reveal that the patient has suffered from alcoholism for several years, although it has not interfered with her work. The patient should be admitted and treated for acute hepatitis while being observed for alcohol withdrawal. Importantly, given the likelihood of cirrhosis, the patient probably has chronic liver disease with an acute-on-chronic alcoholic hepatitis at this time. In all patients with cirrhosis, infection should be ruled out with blood cultures, chest X-ray, urinalysis/culture, and a diagnostic paracentesis (if ascites is present). This is important because oral steroids can be given to treat acute alcoholic hepatitis. A value greater than 32 on Maddrey's discriminant function (which takes the prothrombin time and total bilirubin into account) indicates that treatment with oral steroids may be of benefit.

Clinical pearls

- The typical biochemical pattern of acute alcoholic hepatitis includes an AST to ALT ratio higher than 2:1, elevated bilirubin levels (if active hepatitis), and elevated GGT levels. In addition, macrocytic anemia and thrombocytopenia are common. Even in those without cirrhosis, alcoholics commonly exhibit thrombocytopenia because of toxicity and bone marrow suppression.
- Other causes of acute hepatitis and jaundice need to be ruled out to make the diagnosis of alcoholic hepatitis and chronic alcoholic liver disease. Definitive diagnosis involves liver biopsy, which may show Mallory's hyaline, ballooning degeneration, and steatosis, among other features.

Impress your attending

How long are steroids given and at what dose?

Treatment with steroids is usually for 4 weeks, followed by a taper. The typical dose is prednisone 40mg daily orally. Treatment is often stopped after a week if no improvement in the bilirubin level and/or prothrombin is detected. A response to steroids can be objectively calculated with a Lille scoring model.

What else is highly important in treating alcoholic hepatitis?

A high caloric intake is vital in recovery, and is often achieved with nasojejunal feeding in patients with severe alcoholic hepatitis.

Case 28

A 35-year-old man presents to his primary-care physician with fatigue. He has felt constantly tired for the past 6 months. He sleeps approximately 8 hours every night. He works as an accountant and finds himself too weak to perform his duties. He denies syncope, or cardiovascular or respiratory symptoms.

Further questioning reveals at least two episodes of diarrhea almost every day for the past 3 months. The stool is foul-smelling and thick in character. The patient denies blood in his stool. He occasionally feels bloated, and has mild periumbilical abdominal pain that is somewhat relieved after bowel motions. He used to suffer from constipation and started a stool softener, which he stopped once the diarrhea started. He admits to 10 lbs of unintentional weight loss over the past 2 months.

The patient lives alone, does not smoke, and only occasionally drinks alcohol. He recently ended a relationship and has felt slightly depressed since then. No symptoms of major depression are present. He denies illicit drug use. The patient's past medical and surgical histories are unremarkable apart from childhood asthma and eczema. His family history is unknown, as he was adopted.

What is your differential diagnosis?

The differential diagnosis includes colonic neoplasia, hypothyroidism, colitis, celiac disease, and irritable bowel syndrome.

Physical examination

Vitals Temperature 99.2°F, HR 60 bpm, BP 110/70mmHg, oxygen saturation 99% on RA.

GEN No obvious distress.

Hands No clubbing or palmar erythema.

HEENT Anicteric, moist mucous membranes, no ulceration. No lymphadenopathy.

CVS Normal S1, S2. No murmurs, rubs, or gallops.

RESP Clear to auscultation.

ABD Soft and non-tender. No hepatosplenomegaly appreciated. Bowel sounds are normal.

Skin No spider angiomas. No other rash or abnormal skin changes noted.

NEURO Alert and oriented to time/place/person. Moving all extremities with 5/5 power.

What blood test(s) will you order?

CBC	WBC	$8.0 \times 10^3/\mu L$

	Hemoglobin	10.0g/dL
	Hematocrit	31%
	Platelets	300 x 10^3/μL
CHEM-7	Na	138mEq/L
	K	3.9mEq/L
	Cl	117mEq/L
	Bicarbonate	26mEq/L
	BUN	10mg/dL
	Creatinine	0.8mg/dL
	Glucose	96mg/dL
LFTs	AST	38 units/L
	ALT	45 units/L
	Alkaline phosphatase	105 units/L
	Total bilirubin	0.8mg/dL
INR		1.0
TSH		2.5 mIU/L

Does this change your differential diagnosis?

Yes. The patient's laboratory data reveal anemia and mildly elevated transaminases. Further tests reveal macrocytic anemia with low iron and vitamin B12 levels. Given the anemia, weight loss, and diarrhea, malabsorption is suspected.

How will you manage this patient?

The patient's symptom of fatigue is probably explained by his anemia. The diarrhea he describes is consistent with malabsorption and possibly steatorrhea. The next step is to obtain a tissue transglutaminase antibody level. It is found to be elevated, which is suggestive of gluten enteropathy (celiac disease).

What imaging test will you order?

The next step is to obtain a gastroenterology consultation for an EGD. Before assigning this 35- year-old man to a lifelong gluten-free diet, most experts would feel histologic confirmation of the diagnosis to be prudent. Therefore, a duodenal biopsy must be performed.

The EGD shows the following image (Figure 66).

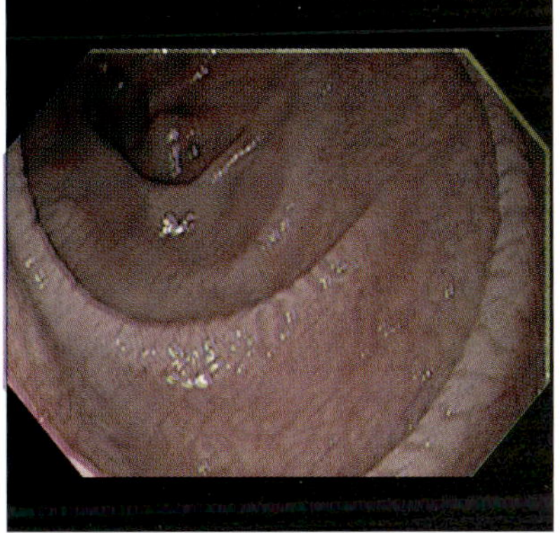

Figure 66.

Describe what you see and read on

This is an endoscopic photo of the duodenum showing scalloping of the mucosal folds and generalized fissuring of the mucosa — the classic endoscopic appearance of celiac disease.

The biopsy confirms villous atrophy and crypt hyperplasia consistent for celiac disease. The treatment is to maintain the patient on a gluten-free diet.

Clinical pearls

- A high index of suspicion is required to diagnose celiac disease in patients with diarrhea, especially if anemia is also present. A family history of chronic diarrhea and anemia should prompt suspicion. Although the tissue transglutaminase antibody test is highly specific, and some experts feel that in the right clinical setting this alone is sufficient for diagnosis, patients (and their primary-care physicians) often insist on a tissue diagnosis before embarking on a lifelong gluten-free diet.

- Anti-tissue transglutaminase antibody and anti-gliadin antibody can rule out celiac disease if the pretest probability of having the disease is low. Anti-gliadin antibody has a high false-positive rate and has largely been replaced by the anti-tissue transglutaminase antibody.
- A false-negative antibody assay can be caused by gluten avoidance. This test can be used on follow-up as a marker of adherence to a gluten-free diet.
- The incidence of celiac disease is at least 1:100 in those of Northern European ancestry.

Impress your attending

What other conditions are associated with celiac disease?

Dermatitis herpetiformis, IgA deficiency, Down's syndrome, and type 1 diabetes mellitus.

How is the severity of celiac disease graded?

The Marsh classification is a histological grading system based on the degree of intraepithelial lymphocytes, villous atrophy, and crypt hyperplasia.

What malignancies are associated with celiac disease?

T-cell lymphoma and small-bowel adenocarcinoma.

Case 29

A 39-year-old man is admitted to hospital with a 4-week history of fever, chills, and night sweats. The previous night the patient's wife measured her husband's temperature at 103°F and says he was shaking all over. The patient has also noticed lower-body muscle aches and complains of mild right upper quadrant abdominal pain. He describes the pain as a dull, constant pain that is slightly worse on inspiration. One week ago he had non-bloody diarrhea that lasted for 3 days. He denies nausea, vomiting, or other GI symptoms. He has not noticed dark urine, pale-colored stools, or jaundice. He denies respiratory, cardiovascular, or neurological symptoms.

There is no history of anorexia or weight loss, none of the patient's contacts are unwell, and he has not traveled recently. The patient's past medical history is significant for type 2 diabetes, which is poorly controlled despite metformin. The patient has smoked 10 cigarettes each day for the past 20 years. He also drinks a few beers every day. He does not have any tattoos and has never received a blood transfusion. He lives with his wife.

What is your differential diagnosis?

The differential diagnosis includes cholecystitis, gastroenteritis, liver abscess, and acute hepatitis.

Physical examination

Vitals Temperature 102.3°F, HR 121 bpm, BP 106/50mmHg, oxygen saturation 96% on RA.

GEN Appears somewhat unwell.

HEENT Anicteric. Moist mucous membranes. No lymphadenopathy.

CVS Normal S1, S2. No additional heart sounds or murmurs.

RESP Clear to auscultation.

ABD Mild right upper quadrant tenderness. Negative Murphy's sign. No hepatosplenomegaly. No masses. Bowel sounds present. Rectal examination reveals guaiac-negative stool.

EXT No edema.

Does this narrow your differential diagnosis?

Yes. The physical examination finding of mild right upper quadrant tenderness without a positive Murphy's sign makes acute cholecystitis less likely.

What blood test(s) will you order?

CBC	WBC	16.9 x10³/μL
	Hemoglobin	13.0g/dL
	Hematocrit	38%
	Platelets	426 x 10³/μL
CHEM 7	Na	139mEq/L
	K	4.1mEq/L
	Cl	106mEq/L

	Bicarbonate	27mEq/L
	BUN	13mg/dL
	Creatinine	1.1mg/dL
	Glucose	408mg/dL
LFTs	AST	20 units/L
ALT		31 units/L
	Alkaline phosphatase 61 units/L	
	Total bilirubin	0.3mg/dL
INR		1.1
Lipase		31 units/L
Lactate		1.3mmol/L
Albumin		2.3g/dL

What is the significance of a low albumin level?

Serum albumin can be low in systemic diseases such as liver cirrhosis or in generalized illness with malnutrition. In addition, acute inflammatory states and certain infections such as liver abscess are also associated with this laboratory abnormality.

The patient should have blood cultures drawn, be started on broad-spectrum antibiotics, and undergo basic imaging.

What imaging test will you order?

A CT scan of the abdomen and pelvis is obtained (Figure 67).

Describe what you see and read on

An axial image through the liver with IV contrast demonstrates an irregular hypodense lesion with peripheral enhancement in the anterior segment of the right hepatic lobe (white arrow). Given the patient's clinical history, this is concerning for an abscess

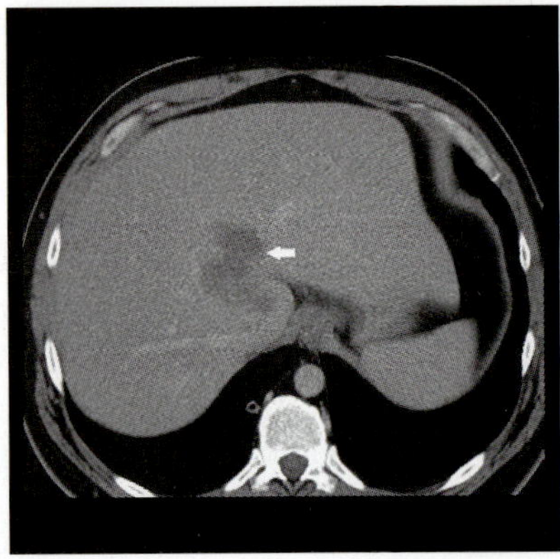

Figure 67.

Given the findings, how will you proceed?

The patient needs to undergo drainage of the abscess by interventional radiology.

Because an infection was suspected on initial presentation, a full work-up was performed including blood cultures. The patient was started on broad-spectrum antibiotics for Gram-negative and anaerobic coverage. The blood cultures grew *Streptococcus anginosus (S. milleri)* group. Serologies were negative for *Entamoeba histolytica* (antibody), and *Echinococcus* antibody was also negative. To look for a possible source, a transthoracic echocardiogram should be performed to rule out cardiac vegetations. Tuberculosis should also be ruled out. Finally, this patient should go on to have a formal dental examination, since poor oral hygiene is a risk factor for hematogenous spread.

Clinical pearls

- Most liver abscesses (80%) are pyogenic (i.e., caused by enteric organisms, anaerobes), but other infections are also possible (e.g.,

Streptococcus, Staphylococcus species). Only a minority are caused by amebic or fungal organisms.

- The source of the infection can be portal bacteremia (e.g., bowel leakage, peritonitis), biliary infection, a surgical wound, or hematogenous spread.
- Treatment includes antibiotics, but abscesses almost always require drainage. This can be via percutaneous needle drainage, which may require placement of a percutaneous catheter.

Impress your attending

What other route of drainage has been reported for hepatic abscesses? Via endoscopic ultrasound.

Case 30

A 62-year-old man presents to the emergency room with 2 days of fevers (up to 104.1°F), chills, and right upper quadrant abdominal pain. He describes the pain as constant but with increases in waves, and rates it as 10/10 at maximal severity. It is accompanied by nausea and the patient is unable to eat or drink. He denies dark urine, pale stools, or changes in his bowel motions.

The patient underwent an orthotopic liver transplant 5 years ago for end-stage liver disease from alcoholic cirrhosis. His course was complicated by hepatic artery thrombosis at the end of the first month after liver transplantation, which was treated with interventional radiology. Thereafter, the patient developed recurrent cholangitis. He has undergone several ERCP procedures including sphincterotomy and removal of biliary sludge. His last bout of cholangitis was a month ago, for which he was treated empirically with ampicillin/sulbactam. He is now taking doxycycline for prophylaxis. The patient's current medications also include metoprolol, simvastatin, tacrolimus, and mycophenolate mofetil.

Physical examination

Vitals	Temperature 100.5°F, HR 88 bpm, BP 110/70mmHg, oxygen saturation 98% on RA.
GEN	No obvious distress.
HEENT	Anicteric. Moist mucous membranes.
CVS	Normal S1, S2. No murmurs, rubs, or gallops.
RESP	Clear to auscultation.
ABD	Soft and non-tender. No right upper quadrant tenderness. No rebound. No hepatomegaly. Bowel sounds normal.
EXT	No edema.

What blood test(s) will you order?

CBC	WBC	7.1 x 10^3/μL
	Hemoglobin	8.5g/dL
	Hematocrit	27.6%
	Platelets	204 x 10^3/μL
CHEM-6	Na	138mEq/L
	K	4.6mEq/L
	Cl	108mEq/L
	Bicarbonate	18mEq/L
	BUN	27mg/dL
	Creatinine	1.4mg/dL
LFTs	AST	49 units/L
	ALT	36 units/L
	Alkaline phosphatase (baseline 200-300 units/L)	432 units/L
	Total bilirubin	0.9mg/dL

Given this patient's history, what empiric management will you start?

Blood cultures should be drawn prior to starting the patient on antibiotics targeted for cholangitis.

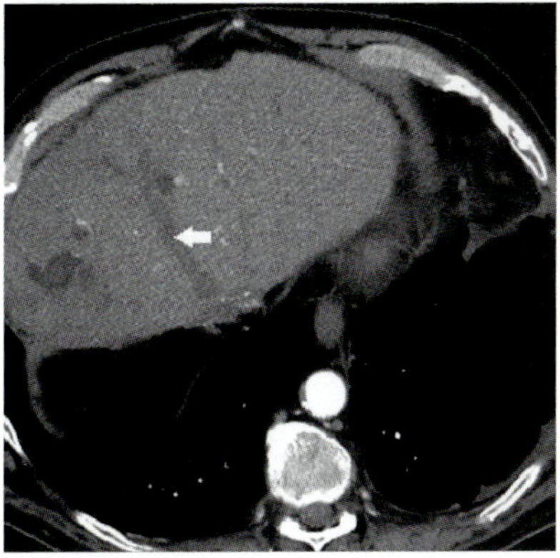

Figure 68.

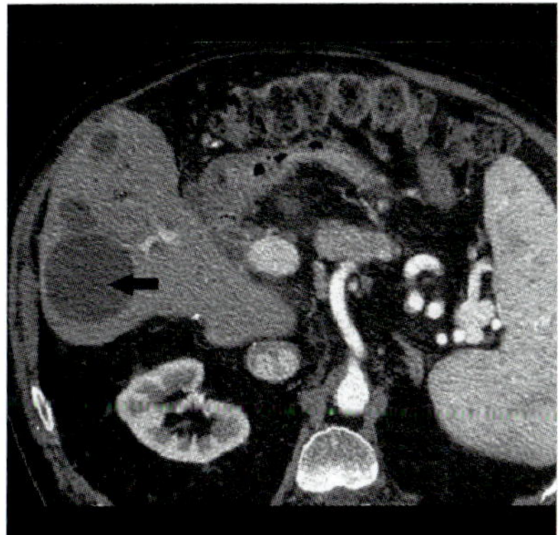

Figure 69.

What imaging test will you order?

A CT scan of the abdomen and pelvis with contrast is obtained (Figures 68 and 69).

Describe what you see and read on

A CT scan of the abdomen with IV contrast is obtained. Multiple axial images through the liver demonstrate dilated intrahepatic biliary ducts (white arrow), with a large hypodense lesion inferiorly in the right hepatic lobe representing a large fluid collection (black arrow). Smaller fluid collections are also identified.

The next step is to perform an ERCP.

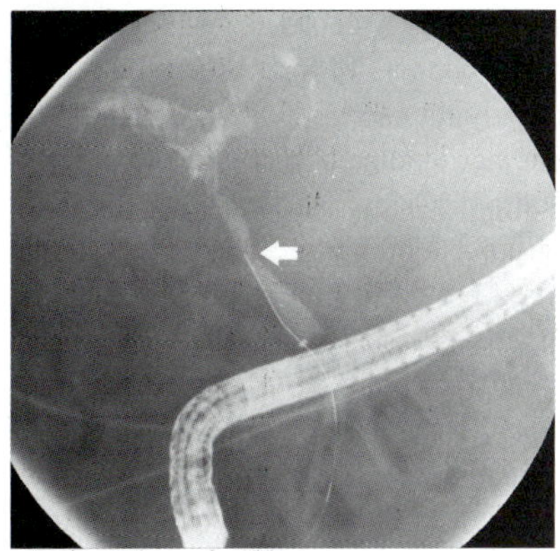

Figure 70

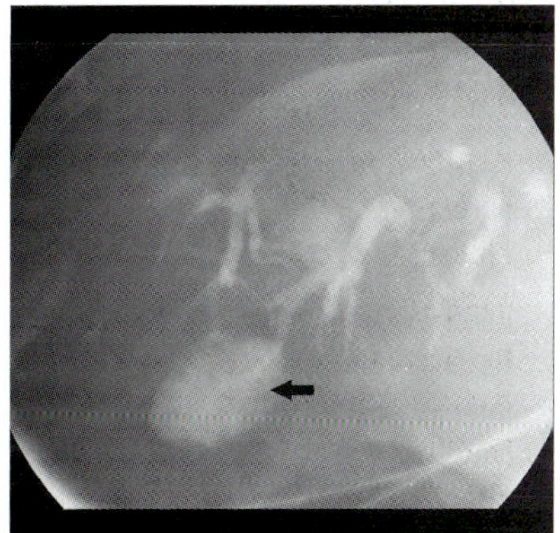

Figure 71.

Images from the procedure are shown in Figures 70 and 71.

Describe what you see and read on

Two fluoroscopic images from the ERCP are shown. Figure 70 shows a stricture in the proximal common bile duct (white arrow). Dilatation of the intrahepatic ducts is also noted. Figure 71 shows dilated ducts as well as a large fluid collection, representing a biloma or abscess (black arrow).

What is the pathophysiology and how will you manage this patient?

The patient has chronic ischemic strictures of the biliary tree and his CT scan shows a biliary collection, known as a biloma. Chronic stricturing and cholangitis can result in biliary epithelial damage leading to bilomas. Bilomas can contain bacteria and may become foci of infection. Large biliary collections may require percutaneous drainage. Strictures and subsequent recurrent cholangitis can be a complication of biliary ischemia. In this patient, biliary ischemia and resulting biliary damage resulted from prior hepatic artery thrombosis. The treatment of choice is percutaneous drainage of the biloma along with antibiotics.

Clinical pearls

- If suspected as a source of infection, a biloma requires percutaneous drainage.
- Bilomas, similar to 'bile lakes,' can be a result of biliary ischemia or iatrogenic biliary tree damage (e.g., caused by ERCP or percutaneous intervention).
- Recurrent cholangitis often requires long-term prophylactic antibiotics aimed at targeting Gram-negative organisms.
- Hepatic artery thrombosis is the second most common cause of liver graft failure (after primary non-function) in the acute setting (within a month of liver transplantation). It is treated with revascularization, retransplantation, or observation.

Impress your attending

What is the definitive treatment for bilomas in this patient?

Liver transplantation.

Case 31

A 63-year-old man presents to the emergency room with abdominal pain. The pain began 4 days ago and has been increasing in severity. The pain was initially generalized but is now located in the left lower quadrant. It is cramping in nature and the patient rates it as 7/10 in severity. He had a few loose stools 2 days ago, but says they were not bloody. He has also noticed a fever at home of 104°F. He has a poor appetite, but no nausea or vomiting.

The patient's past medical history includes constipation, hemorrhoids, and hypertension, for which he is currently taking medications. He is retired and lives with his wife. He does not drink alcohol or smoke. He has not traveled recently and all of his contacts are well.

Physical examination

Vitals Temperature 102.0°F, HR 115 bpm, BP 100/60mmHg, oxygen saturation 98% on RA.

GEN Appears to be distressed.

HEENT Moist mucous membranes. No scleral icterus. No lymphadenopathy.

CVS Normal S1, S2. No murmurs, rubs, or gallops.

RESP Clear to auscultation.

ABD Tender to palpation in left lower quadrant. No rebound or guarding. Bowel sounds are present. Rectal examination reveals guaiac-negative stool.

EXT No clubbing or edema.

What blood test(s) will you order?

CBC	**WBC**	14.5 x 10^3/μL
	Hemoglobin	14g/dL
	Hematocrit	39%
	Platelets	460 x 10^3/μL

CHEM-7, amylase, lipase, and LFTs are all within normal limits.

What is the most likely diagnosis?

The patient has pain in the left lower quadrant, with fever and leukocytosis. In addition he has a history of constipation, which is the probable cause of his hemorrhoids. The most likely diagnosis is diverticulitis, although a diverticular abscess cannot be ruled out

What imaging test will you order?

CT scans of the abdomen and pelvis are obtained (Figures 72 and 73).

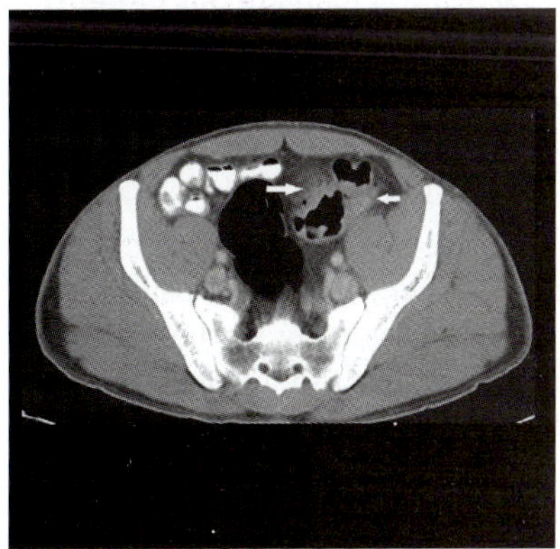

Figure 72. *Image Coutesy of Dr. Steve Allen.*

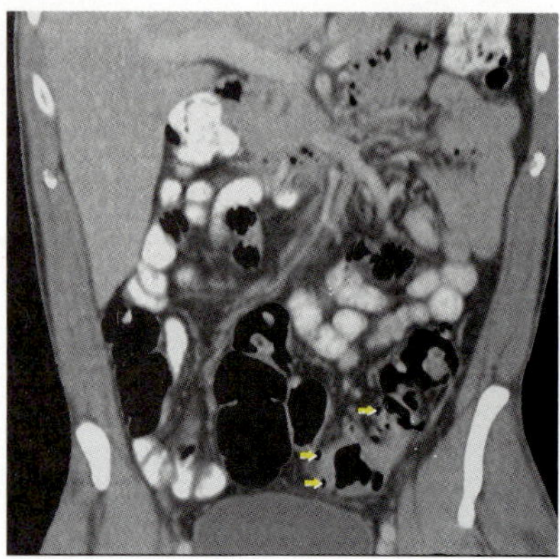

Figure 73. *Image Coutesy of Dr. Steve Allen.*

Describe what you see and read on

CT axial (Figure 72) and coronal (Figure 73) images are obtained of the abdomen and pelvis through the level of the sigmoid colon. Both oral and IV contrast have been administered. Numerous diverticula (yellow arrows) are noted with extensive fat stranding and adjacent inflammatory changes (white arrows) in the mesentery. No discrete fluid collection, focal contained perforation, or pneumoperitoneum is seen. The findings are consistent with uncomplicated diverticulitis of the sigmoid colon.

How will you manage this patient?

Given that the severity of the pain has increased over the past few days, the patient should be admitted to hospital and immediately started on IV antibiotics for Gram-negative and anaerobic organisms. The patient does not show physical or biochemical signs of dehydration, so IV fluids are not currently required. Because the patient's condition has been ongoing for at least 4 days and he was eating at home, it is reasonable to let him continue to eat — he need not be nil by mouth. The patient will improve in the next 24¬ 48 hours, when he can be safely discharged with a course of oral antibiotics.

Clinical pearls

- Diverticulitis can be complicated by perforation, peritonitis, and abscess formation. These should be excluded, as they may require surgical treatment.
- Diverticular bleeding can be significant and should be managed aggressively when it occurs.
- Some cases may be managed in the outpatient setting. As a general rule, patients with fever, leukocytosis, older age, and multiple comorbidities should be treated as an inpatient with IV antibiotics.
- Recurrent attacks of diverticulitis, particularly with complications, may warrant surgical resection of the involved segment of the colon.
- Colonoscopy is contraindicated in acute diverticulitis.

Impress your attending

What procedure should patients undergo on an outpatient basis after treatment for acute diverticulitis?

A colonoscopy should be performed to visualize the extent of the diverticulosis and rule out a perforating carcinoma, which can have a similar clinical presentation and appearance on CT.

Case 32

A 64-year-old man is admitted after suffering an apparent syncopal episode while doing sit-ups. He reports no fever, chills, sweats, jaundice, abdominal pain, nausea, vomiting, diarrhea, or constipation, but has lost 30 lbs in weight during the last 6 months. His past medical history is notable for hyperlipidemia, hypertension, and petit mal seizures. He is a social drinker with occasional binges; he quit smoking 10 years ago. There is no family history of GI disorders of any kind.

Physical examination

Vitals Temperature 97.2°F, HR 80 bpm, BP 132/88mmHg, oxygen saturation 98% on RA.

GEN A well-nourished, well-developed white man in no obvious distress.

HEENT Moist mucous membranes. No scleral icterus. No cervical adenopathy.

CVS Normal S1, S2. No murmurs, rubs, or gallops.

RESP Clear to auscultation.

ABD Soft, non-tender, and non-distended. Normal bowel sounds are present. There is no appreciable mass or hepatosplenomegaly. Rectal examination shows no masses and heme-negative brown stool.

EXT No clubbing, cyanosis, or edema.

Skin No jaundice, spider angiomas, rash, or bruising.

What imaging test will you order?

The patient undergoes a CT angiography of the chest for other indications. Although there is no finding in the chest, an abnormality is found at the most caudal images of the CT angiogram (Figure 74).

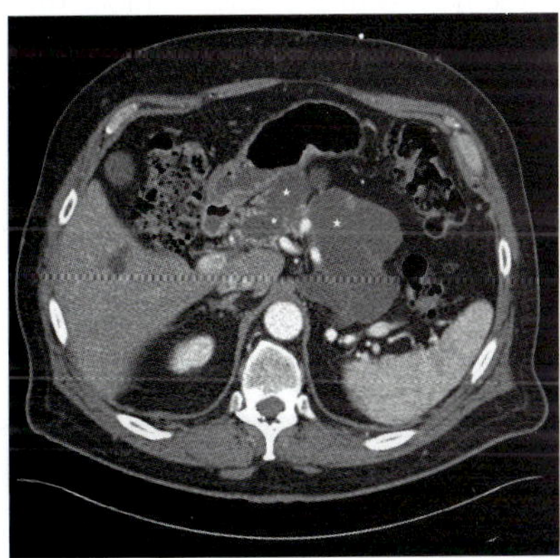

Figure 74.

Describe what you see and read on

Figure 74 shows an axial image of the most inferior image obtained during CT angiography. It shows a markedly dilated dorsal pancreatic duct (white stars), essentially replacing the body and tail of the pancreas. Little if any pancreatic parenchyma is visible.

How will you proceed?

This is an older man who is essentially asymptomatic but was found to have marked dilation of the dorsal pancreatic duct on a CT scan. Although the patient has a fairly significant history of alcohol use, he has no pancreatic calcifications, no history of acute or recurrent pancreatitis, and no abdominal pain, making a diagnosis of chronic pancreatitis unlikely. A post-traumatic benign stricture can cause proximal pancreatic duct enlargement, but these are usually seen in the midline years after a blunt abdominal trauma that compresses the pancreas against the spine.

A neoplasm is far more likely. A pancreatic ductal adenocarcinoma of the very distal ductal system, situated right before the ampulla, could cause obstruction of the duct with proximal dilation. This obstruction would be gradual in onset and could be expected to be painless, as is often the case in pancreatic cancer. However, one would expect a lesion in the most distal pancreatic duct to also cause biliary obstruction. This patient's bilirubin and LFTs are normal and the biliary tree is not dilated on the CT scan, making this diagnosis unlikely as well.

A cystic neoplasm of the pancreas would not be expected to be multiloculated as seen here (the entire pancreas appears to be replaced by cystic structures). Rather, cystic pancreatic neoplasms usually form solitary round or oval lesions. This leaves only one plausible diagnosis: an intraductal papillary mucinous neoplasm (also termed an intraductal mucinous pancreatic tumor).

What imaging test will you now order?

An MRI of the abdomen is obtained for further evaluation (Figure 75).

Describe what you see and read on

Single axial and coronal T2 HASTE images are shown. The pancreas is markedly abnormal. It appears to be comprised mostly of a markedly distended main pancreatic duct (black stars), most severely dilated in the tail, measuring up to 5cm in width. There are no distinct intraluminal filling defects to indicate the presence of a stone. Although not demonstrated on these images, the biliary tree is normal.

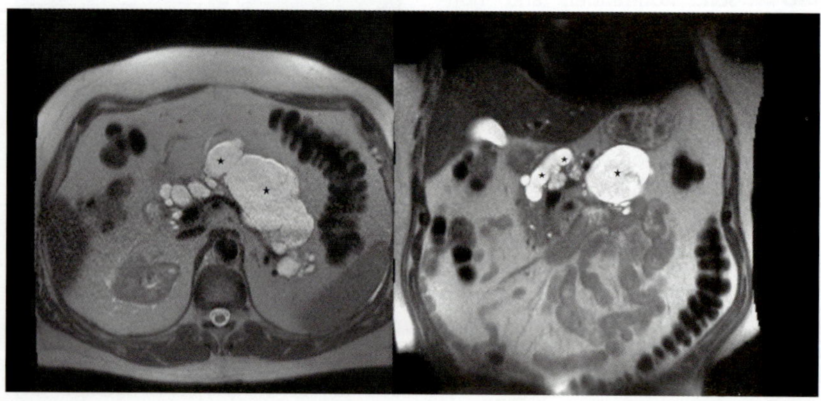

Figure 75.

What is the most likely cause, and what further testing is needed?

The MRI findings are most consistent with an intraductal papillary mucinous neoplasm. An ERCP is performed in an attempt to confirm the radiologic diagnosis. An endoscopic photo from that procedure is shown in Figure 76.

Describe what you see and read on

The major papilla has a gaping os, which is filled with mucus. This finding is pathognomonic of intraductal papillary mucinous neoplasm. This large orifice was easily cannulated and injected with contrast, which revealed a main pancreatic duct that was dilated throughout and filled with mucin.

What additional studies are needed ?

Treatment is surgical, and it would be wise to locate the source of the mucinous neoplasm before the operation. Although some intraductal papillary mucinous neoplasms are described as multifocal, this is often based on the presence of two or more small cystic lesions seen in the pancreas on cross-sectional imaging and is usually without pathologic confirmation. Therefore, the true incidence of multifocal disease is unknown. Most lesions of the type that fill the main pancreatic duct with mucin (as seen here) are unifocal, and the surgeon must determine whether the lesion is to the left or the right of the superior mesenteric artery and vein in order to guide surgical management.

This patient underwent upper endoscopic ultrasound. This located a 5-6mm papillary excrescence in the dorsal duct in the tail of the pancreas. This was suspected to be the papillary neoplasm. Because of intervening blood vessels, fine-needle aspiration was not possible. No suspicious lymph nodes were detected.

The patient went to surgery, where the surgeon bisected the pancreas in the region of the superior mesenteric vein. By passing a ureteroscope both proximally and distally, the surgeon was able to determine that the small papillary lesion in the tail was the only abnormality. A distal pancreatectomy was performed, with removal of the tail and most of the body of the gland. Pathologic evaluation showed a unifocal intraductal papillary mucinous neoplasm in the tail with clean resection margins.

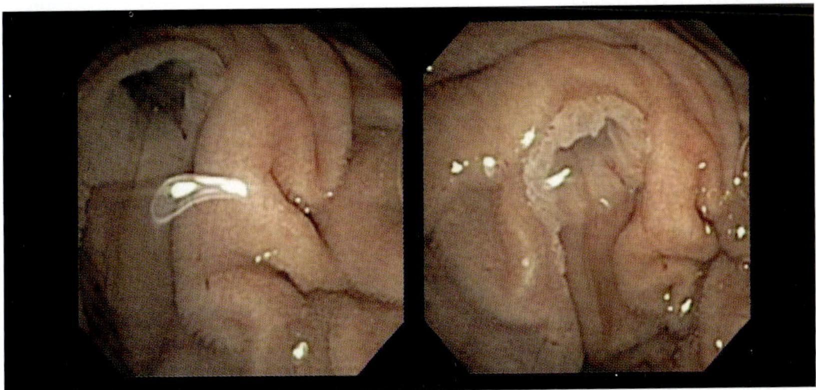

Figure 75.

Clinical pearls

- Patients with an intraductal papillary mucinous neoplasm can present with jaundice, pain, weight loss, vomiting, or pancreatitis. However, the condition is usually asymptomatic and detected incidentally.
- Intraductal papillary mucinous neoplasms are felt to be precancerous neoplasms, but the frequency of malignant transformation is unknown. Treatment is therefore surgical.
- Prior to surgery, one must attempt to locate the mucus-secreting intraductal lesion. This can be challenging. Endoscopic ultrasound and other cross-sectional imaging modalities are often used. It is also wise to look for evidence of multifocality prior to surgery. Multifocality mandates either total pancreatectomy or more intensive surveillance.
- Postoperative surveillance after resection is a controversial topic, with no agreed-upon guidelines for surveillance interval or imaging modality.

Impress your attending

What is the natural history of untreated intraductal papillary mucinous neoplasm?

Although these neoplasms are generally benign when first discovered, they may eventually undergo malignant transformation, becoming an adenocarcinoma or a mucinous adenocarcinoma.

What other imaging modality not already mentioned can sometimes be used to isolate the papillary lesion in this disease?

Pancreatoscopy, using a 'mother/daughter' scope at ERCP, can sometimes be used to identify the neoplastic focus in the pancreatic duct by direct visualization.

Intraductal papillary mucinous neoplasms are usually grouped together with cystic neoplasms of the pancreas. What are the other cystic neoplasms?

Serous cystadenoma (also called microcystic adenoma), mucinous cystadenoma (also called macrocystic adenoma), mucinous cystadenocarcinoma, solid pseudopapillary neoplasm, and pancreatic neuroendocrine tumors that undergo central necrosis with cystic change.

Case 33

A 48-year-old Chinese man presents to your clinic with a 2-month history of vague right upper quadrant pain. The pain is described as dull and achy. The patient rates it as 2/10 in severity and says it is non-radiating. He also describes a sense of tightness in his abdomen and feels his abdomen is growing in size. There are no relieving or exacerbating factors.

The patient also has felt fatigued and is unable to perform his usual daily activities. He has no appetite and has unintentionally lost more than 10 lbs in body weight over the past 4 months. He recently emigrated from China and has not seen a physician for more than 20 years. He is currently working as a chef. He is not on any medications and has no past medical or surgical history. He denies taking herbal remedies or over-the-counter medications. He has not experienced nausea, vomiting, or altered bowel motions.

What is your differential diagnosis?

The differential diagnosis includes ascites, chronic hepatitis, cirrhosis, colorectal cancer, GI malignancy, and hepatocellular carcinoma.

On further questioning, the patient says he was once told he had hepatitis, but never received treatment.

Physical examination

Vitals	Temperature 98.0°F, HR 70 bpm, BP 130/80mmHg, oxygen saturation 98% on RA.
GEN	No obvious distress.
HEENT	Moist mucous membranes. No scleral icterus. No lymphadenopathy.
CVS	Normal S1, S2. No murmurs, rubs, or gallops.
RESP	Clear to auscultation.
ABD	Tender to palpation in right upper quadrant, with two-fingerbreadth hepatomegaly below the right costal margin. Splenomegaly is noted. Bowel sounds are normal. Shifting dullness is present. Rectal examination reveals brown, guaiac-negative stool.
EXT	No clubbing or edema.

What blood test(s) will you order?

CBC	WBC	$10.2 \times 10^3/\mu L$
	Hemoglobin	10g/dL
	Hematocrit	30%
	Platelets	70 x 103/μL
CHEM-6	Na	135mEq/L
	K	4.6mEq/L
	Cl	101mEq/L
	Bicarbonate	25mEq/L
	BUN	20mg/dL
	Creatinine	1.1mg/dL
LFTs	AST	100 units/L

	ALT	130 units/L
	Alkaline phosphatase	400 units/L
	Total bilirubin	2.0mg/dL
Albumin		3. 2g/dL
α-Fetoprotein		100,000ng/mL

Diagnostic/therapeutic paracentesis

Given the positive shifting dullness, a diagnostic/therapeutic paracentesis is performed at the bedside. The fluid study results are shown below:

Blood cells	WBC	1,000 cells/mm^3
	RBC	100 cells/mm^3
	Neutrophils	10%
	Monocytes	5%
Gram stain		Negative
Albumin		1.5g/dL
Cytology		Rare mesothelial cells, no malignant cells present

Other blood work

Other blood work returns and shows the following:

Hepatitis B surface antigen	Positive
Hepatitis B surface antibody	Negative
Hepatitis B core IgM	Negative
Hepatitis C antibody	Negative
Hepatitis B DNA quantification	950,000 IU/mL
Hepatitis e-antibody	Negative
Hepatitis e-antigen	Positive

How will you proceed?

The patient clearly has cirrhosis and resulting ascites from portal hypertension (serum-ascites albumin gradient >1.1). His elevated transaminases, e-antigen positivity, and high viral loads suggest a chronic active hepatitis B infection, which has probably led to cirrhosis and the possible development of hepatocellular carcinoma (elevated α-fetoprotein). The patient requires imaging to look for hepatocellular carcinoma.

What imaging test will you order?

A three-phase CT scan of the abdomen is effective for detecting hepatic lesions. The phases obtained are late arterial, portal venous, and delayed images. This allows hepatic lesions to be evaluated based on their enhancement and wash-out characteristics with contrast. Hepatocellular carcinoma classically enhances in the late arterial phase because of its vast neovascularity. Since most of the hepatic blood supply is portal venous, normal liver parenchyma will mainly enhance during the portal venous phase. Classic lesions have late arterial enhancement and wash-out on delayed-phase imaging.

A CT scan of the abdomen is obtained (Figures 77 and 78)

Describe what you see and read on

Axial (Figure 77) and coronal (Figure 78) images during the arterial phase are shown. Multiple hepatic lesions showing late arterial enhancement compared with the remainder of the parenchyma are seen in the right hepatic lobe (white arrows). The surface of the liver has a nodular appearance. Trace perihepatic ascites (black arrow) is noted, which is expected given the patient's recent paracentesis. The findings are consistent with multiple lesions, probably representing malignancy in the setting of cirrhosis.

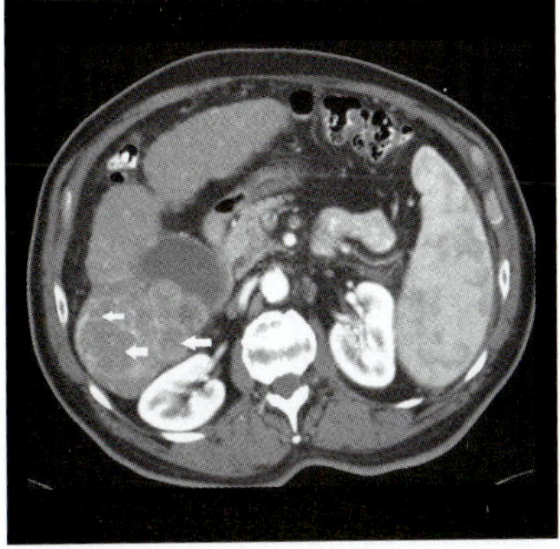

Figure 77.

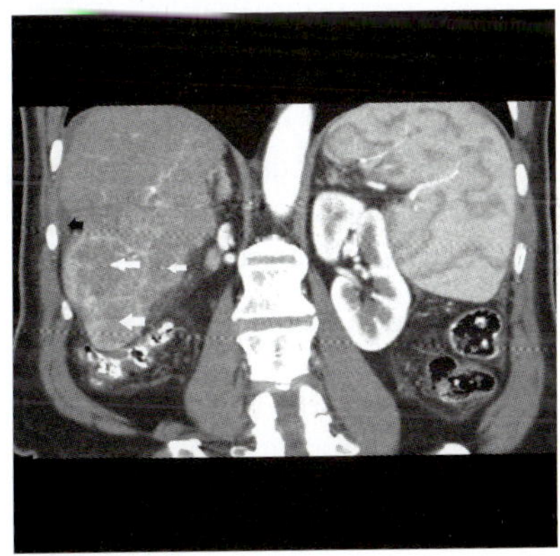

Figure 78.

How will you proceed?

The patient has multiple lesions in his cirrhotic liver. The number and size of his lesions exclude him as a liver transplant candidate. He should be referred to an oncologist for evaluation and palliative measures.

Clinical pearls

- All patients with cirrhosis are at risk of developing hepatocellular carcinoma. These patients should undergo screening every 6 months with abdominal imaging (ultrasound, MRI, or CT scan) and an α-fetoprotein level.
- Chronic hepatitis B infection is an independent risk factor for hepatocellular carcinoma.

Impress your attending

What are the treatment modalities for hepatocellular carcinoma?

- Liver transplant (if within Milan criteria: one mass <5cm in largest diameter, or up to three masses if each <2cm in diameter).
- Locoregional therapies: transarterial catheter embolization, radiofrequency ablation.
- Surgical resection of isolated lesions.
- Chemotherapy: tyrosine kinase inhibitors (e.g., sorafenib).

Case 34

A 47-year-old man with alcoholic cirrhosis presents with 2 days of increasing abdominal pain, which he describes as dull and constant. It is mainly located in the right upper quadrant and epigastric region. The pain is non-radiating. The patient has had no nausea, vomiting, hematemesis, or changes in bowel habit. There are no alleviating or exacerbating factors. He denies fevers, chills, or weight loss.

The patient was diagnosed with alcoholic cirrhosis after a bout of acute alcoholic hepatitis 3 months ago. He was deeply jaundiced, but recovered after a month-long course of oral steroids and alcohol cessation. Since the alcohol cessation the patient's liver function has improved. However, he still has ascites for which he currently takes furosemide and spironolactone. During his prior admission he underwent an upper GI endoscopy, which revealed moderate, non-bleeding, esophageal varices. The varices were not ligated, and he was started on nadolol for primary prophylaxis. The patient's other past medical history is otherwise unremarkable. His father was an alcoholic who died in a car accident. The family history is negative for liver disease of any kind. He lives alone and is a non-smoker. His last alcohol intake was more than 3 months ago.

What is your differential diagnosis?

The differential diagnosis includes cholelithiasis, cholecystitis, spontaneous bacterial peritonitis, gastroenteritis, colitis, hepatic vein thrombosis, and portal vein thrombosis.

Physical examination

Vitals Temperature 98.8°F, HR 55 bpm, BP 114/70mmHg, oxygen saturation 99% on RA.

GEN No obvious distress.

HEENT Moist mucous membranes. No scleral icterus. No lymphadenopathy.

CVS Normal S1, S2. No murmurs, rubs, or gallops.

RESP Clear to auscultation.

ABD Soft and non-tender. Palpable splenomegaly. Minimal shifting dullness. Rectal examination reveals guaiac-negative stool.

EXT No clubbing or edema.

What blood test(s) will you order?

CBC	WBC	8.5 x 10^3/μL
	Hemoglobin	12.7g/dL
	Hematocrit	34%
	Platelets	320 x 10^3/μL
CHEM-7	Na	138mEq/L
	K	4.0mEq/L
	Cl	118mEq/L
	Bicarbonate	24mEq/L
	BUN	40mg/dL
	Creatinine	0.9mg/dL

	Glucose	110mg/dL
LFTs	AST	45 units/L
	ALT	40 units/L
	Alkaline phosphatase	40 units/L
	Total bilirubin	1.5mg/dL
INR		1.3

What other investigations will you perform?

Diagnostic paracentesis and abdominal ultrasound with spectral Doppler imaging. A bedside diagnostic paracentesis is performed and fluid studies are sent.

What other imaging test will you order?

An ultrasound of the abdomen is obtained (Figure 79).

Describe what you see and read on

A single ultrasound image through the main portal vein demonstrates a non-mobile echogenic focus (white arrow). Spectral Doppler imaging demonstrates no flow.

Given these findings, a CT scan of the abdomen and pelvis is obtained (Figure 80).

Describe what you see and read on

An axial CT image of the abdomen with IV contrast during the portal venous phase is shown. The image through the liver shows multiple low- to intermediate-density foci. Many of these are tubular in shape and are within the portal venous system (yellow stars). One of the largest low-density foci has a maximal diameter of 2cm, and measures soft-tissue density (white arrow). Splenic varices are noted (black arrows). Massive splenomegaly is causing compression of the lateral border of the left kidney (black diamond).

Ascitic-fluid study results

Gram stain		Negative
Fluid albumin		0.9mg/dL
Blood cells	WBC	300 cells/mm^3 (20% neutrophils)
	RBC	150 cells/mm^3

How will you proceed?

The radiological findings are suggestive of portal vein thrombosis with cavernous transformation of the main portal vein. The diagnostic paracentesis is negative for spontaneous bacterial peritonitis (>250 cells/mm3 absolute neutrophil count or a positive Gram stain is diagnostic). Portal vein thrombosis can present as a false-positive on Doppler ultrasound, since portal venous stasis can appear similar (turbulent flow). Therefore, portal vein thrombosis should ideally be confirmed with a CT scan of the abdomen, as was done in this case.

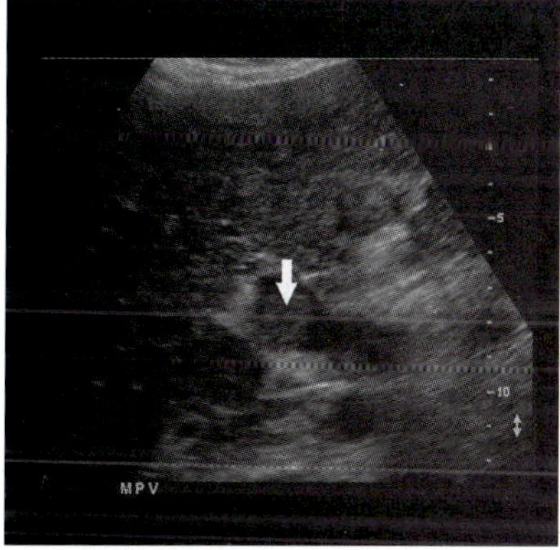

Figure 79. *Image Coutesy of Dr. Jon Cogley.*

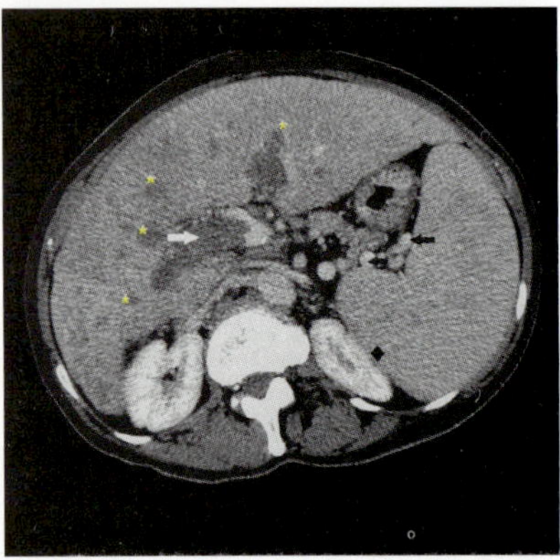

Figure 80. ***Image Coutesy of Dr. Jon Cogley.***

Acute portal vein thrombosis can lead to worsening portal hypertension and is treated with anticoagulation. Most physicians would anticoagulate for 3-6 months. Chronic portal vein thrombosis is characterized by CT findings of cavernous transformation. At this stage, the thrombus is irreversible and anticoagulation has no role. The underlying illness (cirrhosis with portal hypertension) predisposes the patient to thrombosis because of low flow. Anticoagulation is thus ineffective, and engenders only risk without benefit. Therefore, management is with supportive care and treatment of other complications of cirrhosis.

Clinical pearls

- Portal vein thrombosis may occur in patients with cirrhosis. Its incidence increases with worsening liver function.
- The mechanism involves portal venous stasis because of portal hypertension, and acquired deficiencies of anticoagulation factors such as anti-thrombin III.
- The decision to anticoagulate depends on whether the portal vein thrombus is acute or chronic. The risk of bleeding should be balanced with the risk of further clotting. This is difficult to assess in a patient with cirrhosis.

Impress your attending

Does portal vein thrombosis cause ascites?

No, but hepatic vein thrombosis (Budd-Chiari syndrome) may cause ascites because of sinusoidal congestion (post-hepatic portal hypertension).

Case 35

A 48-year-old Chinese man presents to your clinic with a 2-month history of vague right upper quadrant pain. The pain is described as dull and achy. The patient rates it as 2/10 in severity and says it is non-radiating. He also describes a sense of tightness in his abdomen and feels his abdomen is growing in size. There are no relieving or exacerbating factors.

The patient also has felt fatigued and is unable to perform his usual daily activities. He has no appetite and has unintentionally lost more than 10 lbs in body weight over the past 4 months. He recently emigrated from China and has not seen a physician for more than 20 years. He is currently working as a chef. He is not on any medications and has no past medical or surgical history. He denies taking herbal remedies or over-the-counter medications. He has not experienced nausea, vomiting, or altered bowel motions.

Physical examination

Vitals	Temperature 98.2°F, HR 78 bpm, BP 138/88mmHg, oxygen saturation 98% on RA.
GEN	Well-nourished, well-developed African American man in no obvious distress.
HEENT	Pale conjunctivae. Moist mucous membranes. No scleral icterus.
CVS	Normal S1, S2. Faint flow murmur. No rubs or gallops.
RESP	Clear to auscultation.
ABD	Soft and non-tender. No appreciable mass or hepatosplenomegaly. Rectal examination significant for heme-positive brown stool.
EXT	No clubbing, cyanosis, or edema. No palmar erythema.

What blood test(s) will you order?

CBC	WBC	13.0 x 10^3/µL
	Hemoglobin	5.3g/dl
	Hematocrit	19%
	Platelets	426 x 10^3/µL
CHEM-6	Na	143mEq/L
	K	1.9mEq/l
	Cl	107mEq/L
	Bicarbonate	23mEq/L
	BUN	16mg/dL
	Creatinine	1.6mg/dL
LFTs	AST	75 units/L
	ALT	32 units/L
	Alkaline phosphatase	136 units/L
	Total bilirubin	1.0mg/dL
INR		1.1

How will you proceed?

This is an older man with symptomatic

anemia and heme-positive stool. The differential diagnosis includes bone marrow suppression from chronic alcohol use with incidental heme-positive stool from alcohol-associated gastritis, peptic ulcer disease, gastritis, esophagitis, or neoplasm. Given his complaint of constipation, colon cancer should figure highly in the differential diagnosis. Given the patient's vomiting and weight loss, evaluation of the upper GI tract is warranted. Endoscopy is the best next step. At endoscopy, he is found to have a lesion in the stomach (Figure 81).

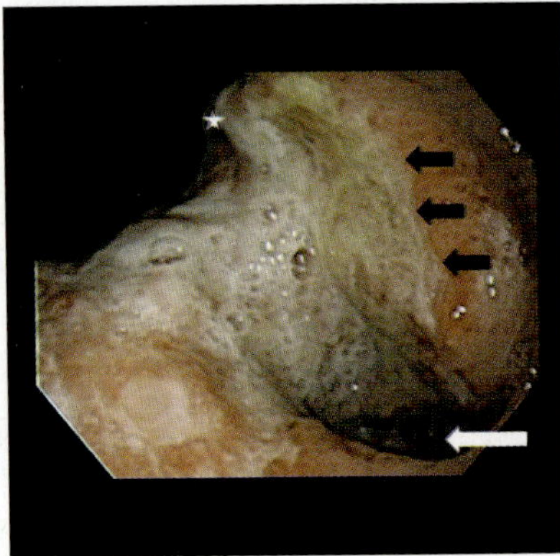

Figure 81.

Describe what you see and read on

This is an endoscopic photo obtained at upper endoscopy. It shows a large ulcerated mass involving the angularis and the antrum. The pylorus is in the distance (white arrow). The partially retroflexed endoscope is visible at the top of the photo (star). The black arrows indicate the edge of the ulcerated mass lesion.

What is the most likely cause and what else should be ruled out?

Adenocarcinoma leads the differential diagnosis list. A large GI stromal tumor is also possible. Lymphoma is in the differential diagnosis list as well, but should be eliminated by the endoscopic biopsies. The lesion is not characteristic of a typical peptic ulcer because of the large size of the mass, the undermining of the edges (which suggests infiltration deep to the mucosa), and the patient's chronic blood loss and anemia. When they bleed, peptic ulcers usually manifest as arterial hemorrhage and not the chronic bleeding seen in this patient, who has not experienced melena, hematemesis, or rectal bleeding. The biopsy results prove this to be a poorly differentiated adenocarcinoma.

What else should be done at the index endoscopy?

If the equipment and expertise are available, an endoscopic ultrasound should also be performed for staging at this time (Figure 82). If suspicious lymph nodes are found, they can be biopsied with fine-needle aspiration. The presence of involved lymph nodes would change the management from resection with curative intent to palliative resection or chemoradiation.

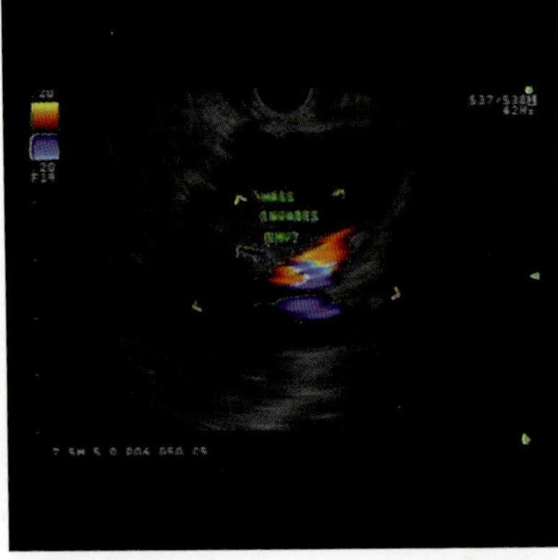

Figure 82.

Describe what you see and read on

Figure 82 shows a heterogeneous and

poorly circumscribed gastric mass extending out beyond the gastric muscularis propria to involve the superior mesenteric artery and vein (color-flow Doppler).

Because the patient has been prepped, and given his marked microcytic anemia, colonoscopy should also be completed to rule out a synchronous neoplasm. A colon cancer metastatic to the stomach is also possible, which is another reason to proceed with colonoscopy.

Clinical pearls

- Gastric cancer can present as iron-deficiency or microcytic anemia. It is often painless.
- Risk factors include alcohol use, smoking, and *Helicobacter pylori* infection.
- Surgery can be curative; chemotherapy and radiation are palliative only.
- Any large gastric ulcer, especially a solitary gastric ulcer, should be biopsied at the index endoscopy to rule out neoplasm. If biopsies are negative, endoscopy should be repeated after 8 weeks of proton-pump inhibitor therapy to ensure healing. An ulcer that persists after 8 weeks of proton-pump inhibitor therapy is highly suspicious for malignancy and should be rebiopsied.

Impress your attending

What are typical sites of metastasis for gastric cancer?

- Gastric adenocarcinoma typically metastasizes to the liver via hematogenous spread from portal venous drainage, and also to local or distant lymph nodes by lymphatic spread. An enlarged, palpable liver or palpable lymph nodes can indicate the diagnosis on physical examination, even before imaging and endoscopy are performed.
- A palpable left supraclavicular lymph node is also called Virchow's node. This is considered a sentinel lymph node for intra-abdominal malignancy, especially gastric cancer.
- The presence of Virchow's node implies the patient has distant metastases and that surgery, if done at all, would be palliative.
- Ovarian malignant lesions from metastatic gastric cancer are called Krukenberg tumors.

Case 36

A 61-year-old woman presents to the emergency room with a 2-day history of bright-red blood per rectum and lower abdominal pain. She has never had these symptoms before. The pain is minimal in the lower abdomen but is mostly present in her rectum as she passes stool. She denies nausea, vomiting, or fever. She is not anorexic and has not lost weight.

The patient is recovering from radiation therapy for cervical cancer, which she underwent 4 months ago. Her other past medical history is significant for hypertension, dyslipidemia, and osteoarthritis. She lives with her husband, and does not smoke or drink alcohol. She had a screening colonoscopy 10 years ago, which was normal. There is no family history of GI disease.

What is your differential diagnosis?

The differential diagnosis includes hemorrhoids, radiation proctitis, infectious proctocolitis, anal fissures, inflammatory bowel disease, and solitary rectal ulcer syndrome.

Physical examination

Vitals Temperature 98.5°F, HR 90 bpm, BP 115/70mmHg, oxygen saturation 99% on RA.

GEN Does not appear significantly distressed.

HEENT Moist mucous membranes. No scleral icterus. No lymphadenopathy.

CVS Normal S1, S2. No murmurs, rubs, or gallops.

RESP Clear to auscultation.

ABD Abdomen is soft and non-tender. No hepatosplenomegaly. Bowel sounds are normal. Rectal examination demonstrates circumferential tenderness and blood-stained stool. No palpable mass.

EXT No clubbing, cyanosis, or edema.

What blood test(s) will you order?

CBC	WBC	9.0 x $10^3/\mu L$
	Hemoglobin	11.5g/dL
	Hematocrit	34%
	Platelets	200 x $10^3/\mu L$
CHEM-7		Normal
LFTs		Normal
INR		1.1

What is the likely diagnosis, and how will you proceed?

Given the patient has recently undergone radiation therapy, she is at risk of radiation proctitis.

The patient continues to have hematochezia. She is admitted for pain control and possible colonoscopy given her history of cervical cancer. The next step is to begin a bowel prep.

Imaging

A colonoscopy is performed the next day. An image obtained during the procedure is shown in Figure 83.

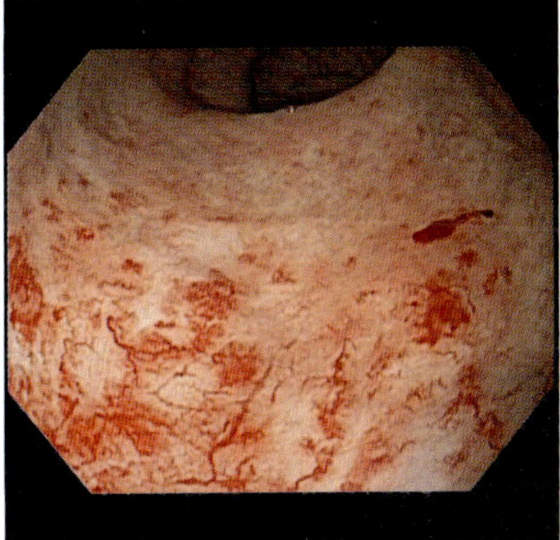

Figure 83.

Describe what you see and read on

This image, obtained at the level of the rectum, shows evidence of twisted, ectatic blood vessels with some oozing. This is consistent with radiation proctitis.

The report says argon plasma coagulation was applied to the vessels, achieving obliteration and hemostasis to the areas of oozing. The patient's symptoms subsided following this procedure and she did not experience further episodes of hematochezia. In addition, her hemoglobin level remained stable.

The plan would be to discharge the patient and perform a sigmoidoscopy 4 weeks later to evaluate the need for repeat argon plasma coagulation.

Clinical pearls

- Radiation proctitis is usually a result of pelvic radiation for prostate or cervical cancer. Hematochezia is the main symptom. Rectal pain or tenesmus, as seen in this patient, is unusual.
- Radiation proctitis can be either acute (within 6 weeks of therapy) or chronic; most cases are chronic. There is no real 'itis' involved. Rather, the manifestations of this syndrome comprise radiation-induced thinning of the mucosa such that the vessels appear to rise to the surface, rupture, and bleed. This generally takes time, which is why most cases occur long after the radiation has been administered.
- The likelihood of developing radiation proctitis appears to be dose-related. There are no good prophylactic treatments.
- Rectal sulfasalazine and steroid preparations along with stool softeners have been used for the medical treatment of radiation proctitis, but these are of dubious utility'. Oral metronidazole has also been trialed, with uncertain effect. The treatment of choice is to ablate the fragile surface vessels with thermal methods, preferably non-contact thermal methods such as argon plasma coagulation or argon ion or Nd:YAG laser. Patients with strictures may need endoscopic balloon dilatation.

Impress your attending

Besides thermal therapy, what other methods can you use to endoscopically control bleeding from proctitis?

- Cryotherapy with liquid nitrogen.
- Additional non-thermal

management includes proctoscopy under anesthesia with application of 4% formalin to the affected mucosa.

Reference

1. Kilig D, Egehan I, Ozenirler S, Dursun A. Double-blinded, randomized, placebo-controlled study to evaluate the effectiveness of sulphasalazine in preventing acute gastrointestinal complications due to radiotherapy. *Radiother Oncol* 2000; 57(2): 125-9.

Case 37

A 55-year-old man is brought into the emergency room by his wife, who found him collapsed in the bedroom. The wife says her husband is a chronic alcoholic who has recently binged after losing his job. However, she thought he seemed well yesterday.

Over the past several months, the patient has become increasingly confused about his normal daily tasks. In addition, his wife has noticed a gradual abdominal swelling. The patient has not sought medical care and does not have a primary-care physician. His wife does not know if he has recently had fevers or chills.

What is your differential diagnosis?

The patient has an altered mental status and fever. The differential diagnosis is broad at this time. His clinical presentation is suggestive of an infectious process. Head trauma and a possible intracranial bleed should also be considered in an alcoholic patient (higher risk of subdural hematoma).

Physical examination

Vitals	Temperature 103.5°F, HR 110 bpm, BP 100/80mmHg, oxygen saturation 95% on RA.
GEN	Anxious, disoriented to place and time. Smells of alcohol.
CVS	Normal S1, S2. No murmurs, rubs, or gallops.
RESP	Bibasilar crackles.
ABD	Distended and tense. A shifting dullness is present. The spleen tip is palpable.
Skin	Palmar erythema. No extremity swelling.
NEURO	Asterixis.

What blood test(s) will you order?

CBC	**WBC**	16.5 x 10^3/µL (90% neutrophils)
	Hemoglobin	10.2g/dL
	Hematocrit	31%
	Platelets	75 x 10^3/µL
CHEM-6	**Na**	130mEq/L
	K	3.5mEq/L
	Cl	99mEq/L
	Bicarbonate	12mEq/L
	BUN	25mg/dL
	Creatinine	2.5mg/dL
LFTs	**AST**	60 units/L
	ALT	55 units/L
	Alkaline phosphatase	212 units/L
	Total bilirubin	2.9mg/dL
Lactate		3.1mmol/L

How would you interpret these data, and how will you proceed?

The patient has leukocytosis with a left shift, increasing the suspicion of infection. Thrombocytopenia is consistent with cirrhosis. Hyponatremia can also occur in the setting of cirrhosis. The patient's renal failure could be acute, but we do not have prior laboratory data. The lactate level can be elevated in the setting of a possible infection and hypoperfusion.

What imaging test will you order?

An ultrasound of the abdomen is obtained (Figure 84).

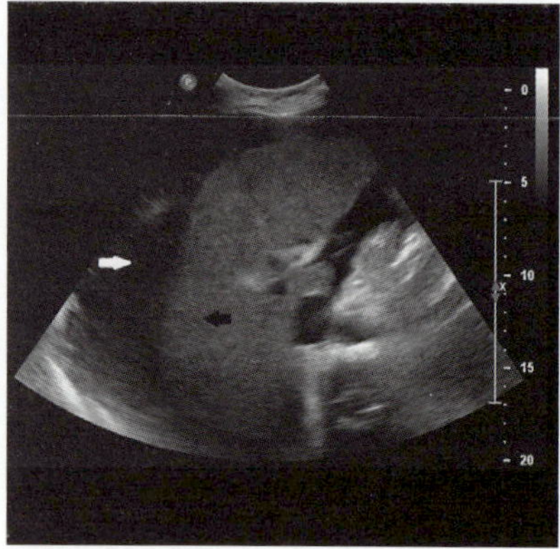

Figure 84.

Describe what you see and read on

This single transverse image through the liver shows a shrunken, nodular-appearing liver (black arrow). The liver has a coarse echotexture. No focal hepatic lesions are seen. A large amount of ascites is present adjacent to the liver (white arrow).

Although not clinically indicated, this patient also undergoes a CT scan of the abdomen and pelvis (Figure 85).

Describe what you see and read on

A single axial slice with oral contrast is shown through the level of the stomach.

There is a massive degree of perihepatic and perisplenic fluid (white arrows), representing massive ascites. The liver is shrunken and has a slight nodular appearance (black arrow). The spleen is generous, but is within normal limits. No varices are seen on this non-intravenous contrast study.

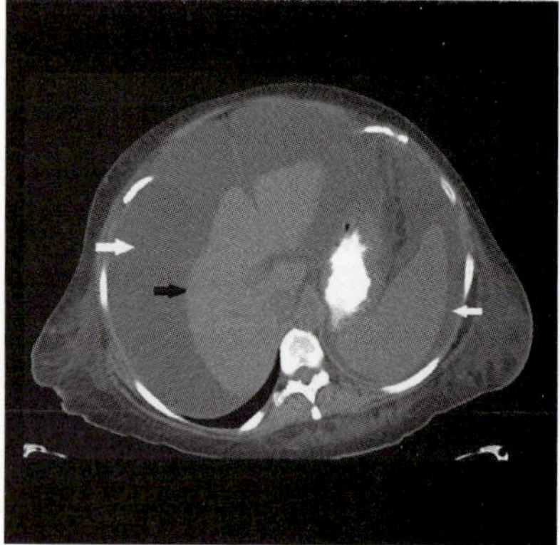

Figure 85.

What is this patient's underlying disease, and what test must you perform?

The patient has cirrhosis, likely alcoholic, and is currently decompensated with ascites and hepatic encephalopathy. An infectious process is probably occurring, which could be triggering the patient's decompensated cirrhosis. Given ascites, spontaneous bacterial peritonitis must be excluded via a diagnostic paracentesis.

A diagnostic and therapeutic paracentesis is performed. A total of 20cc of fluid is initially collected and sent for laboratory assessment. The assessment shows WBC 3000 units/mm3 (90% neutrophils) with minimal blood.

How will you treat the patient?

The patient has spontaneous bacterial peritonitis, characterized by an ascitic neutrophil count of more than 250 cells/mm3. The patient is given 2g of IV ceftriaxone with 1.5g/kg body weight of 25% albumin solution. A Gram stain is pending. The patient should be admitted for further care, preferably to the intensive care unit given his mental status changes/obtundation.

Clinical pearls

- Decompensated cirrhosis can manifest as ascites, hepatic encephalopathy, jaundice, or variceal hemorrhage. The sequelae of portal hypertension can also include hyponatremia and renal failure.
- Spontaneous bacterial peritonitis must be excluded in all patients with cirrhosis and ascites, as this condition can trigger hepatic encephalopathy.
- Spontaneous bacterial peritonitis may be a subclinical presentation, and patients may not exhibit abdominal pain or fever.
- The treatment of spontaneous bacterial peritonitis includes IV third-generation cephalosporin antibiotics and albumin (1.5g/kg body weight on day 1 and 1g/kg body weight on day 3).
- Albumin solution is shown to prevent renal failure, which can occur with spontaneous bacterial peritonitis.

Impress your attending

What are the indications for spontaneous bacterial peritonitis prophylaxis?

Indications include GI bleeding, a prior episode of spontaneous bacterial peritonitis, or ascitic albumin of less than 1g/dL.

Case 38

A 35-year-old man is admitted from the emergency room with a 3-day history of nausea, anorexia, and jaundice. The patient's girlfriend noticed yellowing of his eyes and skin, and encouraged him to go to the hospital. He describes mild abdominal pain located in the right upper quadrant. It is a dull pain without relieving or exacerbating factors. The patient denies diarrhea, constipation, melena, hematemesis, or weight loss.

The past medical history is not significant. The patient had an appendectomy as a child. He has been an IV drug user for the past 5 years and shares needles with his girlfriend. He drinks at least two beers each day. He is currently unemployed and has not traveled outside of the USA recently. He has never received a blood transfusion. He is not on any medications, but takes the occasional acetaminophen for pain. He denies taking acetaminophen or other pain medication in the past few days. He has no history of jaundice.

What is your differential diagnosis?

The differential diagnosis includes acute viral hepatitis, alcoholic hepatitis, choledocholithiasis, acute cholecystitis, and drug-induced toxicity.

Physical examination

Vitals Temperature 99.2°F, HR 75 bpm, BP 125/80mmHg, oxygen saturation 99% on RA.

GEN Appears to be in mild distress.

HEENT Icterus. Moist mucous membranes. No lymphadenopathy.

CVS Normal S1, S2. No murmurs, rubs, or gallops.

RESP Clear to auscultation.

ABD Mild right upper quadrant pain. No guarding or rebound tenderness. No palpable hepatomegaly or splenomegaly.

EXT No clubbing or palmar erythema.

Skin No spider angiomas.

NEURO Alert and oriented to time, place, and person. No asterixis.

What blood test(s) will you order?

CBC	WBC	13 x $10^3/\mu L$
	Hemoglobin	13g/dL
	Hematocrit	38%
	Platelets	350 x $10^3/\mu L$
CHEM-7	Na	135mEq/L
	K	4.2mEq/L
	Cl	114mEq/L
	Bicarbonate	26mEq/L
	BUN	15mg/dL
	Creatinine	1.0mg/dL
	Glucose	98mg/dL
LFTs	AST	1954 units/L
	ALT	2500 units/L

Alkaline phosphatase	190 units/L
Total bilirubin	15.2 units/L
INR	1.3

Does this change your differential diagnosis?

Yes. The patient shows laboratory evidence of acute hepatitis, with AST and ALT levels higher than 1000 units/L. In addition, he has jaundice and a mildly elevated INR. The differential diagnosis for this biochemical picture includes acute viral hepatitis, drug-induced hepatotoxicity or hepatitis, ischemic hepatitis, and autoimmune hepatitis. The very high transaminase levels are inconsistent with alcohol-induced injury, and this can now be excluded. Specific viral serology and other immunologic tests should be requested at this time.

Imaging

The emergency-room physician has ordered an ultrasound of the right upper quadrant (Figure 86).

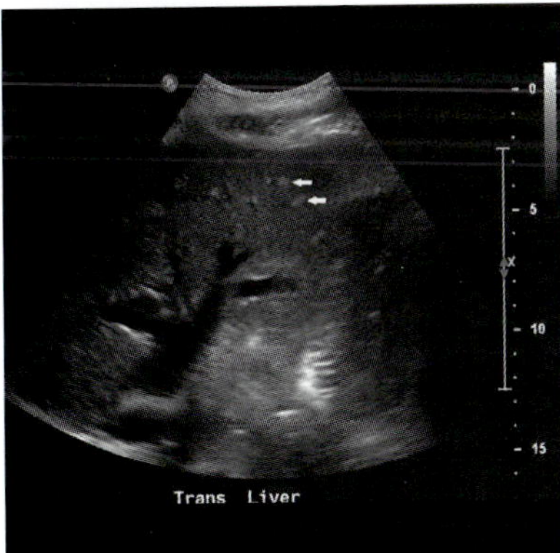

Figure 86.

Describe what you see and read on

This transverse image of the liver obtained with a curved transducer shows tubular areas of increased echogenicity (white arrows) suggestive of the 'starry sky' appearance. These represent prominent portal triads compared with the relatively hypoechoic, edematous hepatic parenchyma. No focal lesions are seen. These findings are suggestive of acute viral hepatitis or hepatic congestion caused by right-sided heart failure.

Further laboratory data

Hepatitis C antibody	Negative
Hepatitis C RNA (quantification)	Negative
Hepatitis B surface antigen	Positive
Hepatitis B surface antibody	Negative
Hepatitis B core IgM antibody	Positive
Acetaminophen level	Undetectable
ANA	1:20
Anti-smooth muscle antibody	1:20
Serum IgG	1500mg/dL

How will you proceed?

Given the ultrasound findings and laboratory data, the patient has an acute hepatitis B infection. This is characterized by his positive hepatitis B surface antigen and IgM core antibody positivity. In addition, the patient has positive risk factors for contraction of the disease. There is no specific treatment at this time and conservative management with fluids is the priority of care.

The patient's mental status remains clear and his INR normalizes to 1.0 within 2 days. His LFTs continue to improve on a daily basis.

Clinical pearls

- Most patients with hepatitis B (up

to 90%) clear the virus and develop hepatitis B surface antibody. Approximately 10% go on to have chronic hepatitis B infection.

- There is no advantage to antiviral therapy for most patients with hepatitis B infection in the acute setting. However, patients with concurrent hepatitis C, HIV, or pre-existing cirrhosis have a poorer outcome and may benefit from treatment for acute hepatitis B.
- The treatment of chronic hepatitis B depends on a variety of factors, including hepatitis B viral load, hepatitis e-antigen/antibody status, and active infection (determined by elevated liver transaminases). In addition, patients with significant liver fibrosis as determined by liver biopsy should be treated for chronic hepatitis B infection.

Impress your attending

Does a negative hepatitis C antibody test rule out acute hepatitis C?

No. The hepatitis C viral load needs to be checked.

Is a liver biopsy needed in patients with acute hepatitis?

For the most part, a biopsy may be useful when autoimmune hepatitis is suspected. It is notoriously difficult to differentiate between acute viral hepatitis and drug-induced hepatitis on biopsy, as both show evidence of diffuse inflammation in the portal and lobular regions.

Autoimmune hepatitis has typical features such as plasma cells and evidence of interface hepatitis. It requires immunosuppression with prednisone and/or a steroid-sparing agent such as azathioprine; therefore, biopsy is needed in cases where autoimmune hepatitis must be distinguished from viral hepatitis.

Our patient has no stigmata of autoimmune hepatitis. In addition, his clinical presentation and numerous risk factors for hepatitis B, and his laboratory results indicating acute hepatitis B infection, obviate the need for liver biopsy.

What are other causes of acute hepatitis and how are they treated?

Ischemic hepatitis is usually seen in patients with severe hypotension, which can be seen in shock. LFTs can rise dramatically but improve when normal hemodynamics are achieved.

The most common cause of drug-induced liver injury is acetaminophen, which can cause an acute rise in LFTs. Importantly, acetaminophen toxicity can lead to acute liver failure. Liver failure results in coagulopathy and encephalopathy, which is why both of these features need to be monitored closely in the intensive care setting. The toxic metabolite of acetaminophen, NADPQI (N-acetyl-p-benzoquinone-imine), accumulates in acute acetaminophen-induced liver failure. N-acetylcysteine counteracts the toxicity of NADPQI, but must be given within hours of the acetaminophen overdose.

Case 39

The gastroenterology service is consulted about a 65-year-old woman on the oncology ward. The patient was discharged to a nursing facility after completing a second cycle of chemotherapy for ovarian cancer, but was readmitted to the oncology service 2 days ago for diarrhea. The diarrhea was initially copious and foul-smelling. She was diagnosed with *Clostridium difficile* in her stool (toxin-positive) and treatment with oral metronidazole was commenced. One week prior, the patient completed a 7-day course of ciprofloxacin for a urinary tract infection that resolved. Over the past 24 hours, she has been febrile to a maximum temperature of 103.5°F and has experienced chills. She has developed moderate to severe crampy abdominal pain in the interim. She continues to pass foul-smelling diarrhea, with up to 10 bowel movements in the past 24 hours.

The patient's past medical history is notable only for hypertension and dyslipidemia. She was diagnosed with ovarian cancer last year, and has undergone resection and omentectomy. There is no history of preceding GI disease. She had a screening colonoscopy in the past that was unremarkable. Current antibiotics include only oral metronidazole. Her family history is negative for colorectal neoplasia and inflammatory bowel disease. The patient does not drink alcohol or smoke cigarettes. She is accompanied by her husband and two children.

What is your differential diagnosis?

The differential diagnosis includes severe *C. difficile* colitis, toxic megacolon, infectious colitis, Ogilvie's syndrome, and recurrent ovarian cancer.

Physical examination

Vitals Temperature 102.10F, HR 110 bpm, BP 105/60mmHg, oxygen saturation 97% on RA.

GEN Cachectic and appears distressed.

Hands No clubbing or palmar erythema.

HEENT Dry mucous membranes. No lymphadenopathy.

CVS Normal S1, S2. No rubs, murmurs, or gallops.

RESP Clear to auscultation bilaterally.

ABD Distended abdomen. Tenderness throughout. No rebound. Increased tympany on percussion throughout. No hepatosplenomegaly appreciated. Bowel sounds are normal. The rectal examination is significant for yellow liquid stool.

Skin No spider angiomas. No rash or abnormal skin changes.

What blood test(s) will you order?

CBC	WBC	29 x 10^3/μL
	Hemoglobin	10g/dL

	Hematocrit	29%
	Platelets	490 x 10^3/μL
CHEM-7	Na	138mEq/L
	K	4.9mEq/L
	Cl	115mEq/L
	Bicarbonate	15mEq/L
	BUN	27mg/dL
	Creatinine	0.8mg/dL
	Glucose	99mg/dL
LFTs	AST	40 units/L
	ALT	45 units/L
	Alkaline phosphatase	116 units/L
	Total bilirubin	0.8mg/dL
	INR	
	Lactate	

Do these findings change your differential diagnosis?

Yes. There is evidence of leukocytosis, which can be seen in *C. difficile* infection. The likelihood of severe *C. difficile* infection and toxic megacolon remains, given the temporal relationship of the patient's diagnosis and clinical deterioration.

What imaging test will you order?

CT scans of the abdomen and pelvis are obtained (Figures 87 and 88).

Describe what you see and read on

Axial (Figure 87) and coronal (Figure 88) images of the abdomen and pelvis are shown. Oral and IV contrast was administered. The colon is diffusely dilated and gas-filled (white arrows). Diffuse mural thickening of the colonic wall is noted (yellow arrows). There is hazy stranding of the pericolic fat (white arrowhead). The cecum measures only 5cm in its maximum dimension. There is no intra-abdominal abscess, and neither pneumatosis nor pneumoperitoneum are seen. A hypodensity appearing to be of fluid attenuation is present in the inferior right lobe of the liver, representing a cyst (yellow asterisk). A small aneurysm of the aorta (red arrow) with a mural thrombus is present, with extensive atherosclerotic calcifications of the aorta.

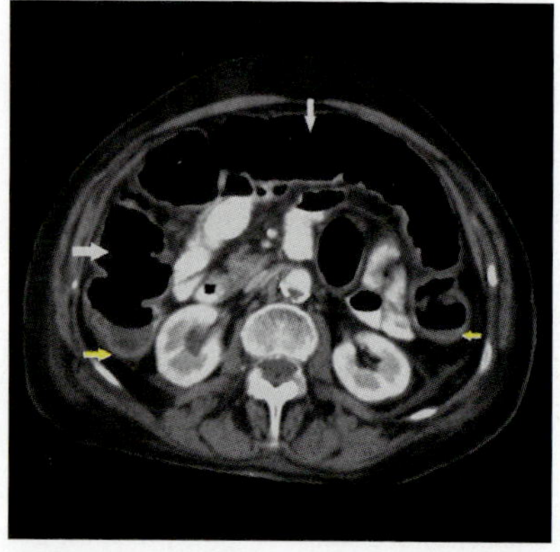

Figure 87.

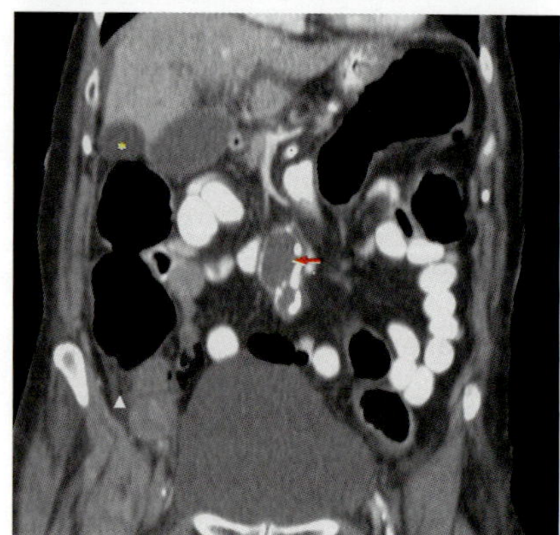

Figure 88.

How will you proceed?

Given the clinical symptoms and CT findings, the patient has severe worsening *C. difficile* infection resulting in toxic megacolon. This diagnosis carries a high morbidity and mortality. The patient is started on oral vancomycin and IV metronidazole for her severe *C. difficile*-associated diarrhea. She is transferred to the intensive care unit, placed on nasogastric suction and given bowel rest. The patient should undergo serial abdominal examinations with repeat imaging if she clinically deteriorates.

Clinical pearls

- *Clostridium difficile* infection is increasingly common in hospitalized and institutionalized patients (e.g., those in nursing homes).
- Recent antibiotic use, particularly clindamycin and fluoroquinolones, is a risk factor.
- Immunosuppressed patients are at a particular risk for developing severe C. difficile¬associated diarrhea.
- Oral vancomycin is becoming an increasing popular treatment for *C. difficile* infection because it is associated with a decreased rate of recurrent disease. Oral vancomycin is preferred over metronidazole for moderate to severe disease. IV metronidazole is combined with oral vancomycin for the treatment of severe *C. difficile*-associated diarrhea (including toxic megacolon).
- Toxic megacolon occurs in the settings of inflammatory bowel disease and infectious colitis such as *C. difficile* infection.
- Perforation is a complication of toxic megacolon. It requires laparotomy and partial or complete colectomy (with ileostomy).
- In the absence of mechanical obstruction or infection/ inflammation, Ogilvie's syndrome (acute colonic pseudo-obstruction) is a possible diagnosis. Ogilvie's syndrome requires conservative treatment including nasogastric suction, bowel rest, and correction of electrolyte imbalances. Colonic decompression can be attempted in some patients if conservative measures fail. However, it is debatable if this changes the course of the disease.

Impress your attending

Is a colonoscopy or sigmoidoscopy warranted if toxic megacolon is suggested?

No. In fact, active inflammation and friable mucosa mean an increased risk of perforation if colonoscopy is performed.

What other causes of toxic megacolon are there?

Complication of inflammatory bowel disease, ischemic colitis, diverticulitis, and volvulus.

Case 40

A 70-year-old woman is brought to the emergency room with shortness of breath after being found at home by her daughter. She was sitting upright on a chair with labored breathing. The emergency medical services found the patient to be hypoxemic with fine crackles throughout all the lung fields. On arrival at the emergency room, the patient is hypotensive with a BP of 90/50mmHg and pulse of 100 bpm. She is afebrile, confused, and unable to complete sentences. She is intubated emergently and started on ventilator support. She is started on dopamine for BP support. The patient undergoes panculture and is given broad-spectrum antibiotics.

Further history reveals the patient has congestive heart failure with an ejection fraction of 30%. She has had a myocardial infarction in the past, and has an implantable cardioverter/defibrillator in situ. This is interrogated but does not show arrhythmia events. The patient is taken to the intensive care unit. While being transported, she has an acute episode of bright-red hematochezia and continues to have two additional large episodes over the next hour. The inpatient GI service is consulted for lower GI bleeding.

Records show the patient had a colonoscopy in the remote past, which was normal. She has had a total abdominal hysterectomy, but otherwise no surgeries. The family history is negative for colorectal neoplasia and inflammatory bowel disease. The social history is negative for alcohol or cigarette intake. Her BP has improved by this time, and diuretics are started for pulmonary edema.

What is your differential diagnosis?

The differential diagnosis includes ischemic colitis, diverticulitis, and infectious colitis. Her mental status changes could be due to sepsis, medications, or metabolic derangement. There is no history of liver disease, and therefore hepatic encephalopathy is not suspected.

Physical examination

Vitals Temperature 97.5°F, HR 90 bpm, BP 100/65mmHg, oxygen saturation 99% on 100% fraction of inspired oxygen, positive end-expiratory pressure 10cmH2O.

Skin/hands No clubbing, palmar erythema, or spider angiomas. No rash or abnormal skin changes noted.

HEENT Pupils equal and reactive to light and accommodation. Moist mucous membranes with no ulceration noted. Nolymphadenopathy.

CVS Normal S1, S2. No murmurs, rubs, or gallops.

RESP Fine crackles to auscultation at the lung bases.

ABD Distended abdomen. Increased tympany to percussion throughout. No hepatosplenomegaly is appreciated. Bowel sounds are normal. Rectal examination reveals bright-red blood present on a gloved finger. No rectal masses are palpable.

NEURO Minimally withdrawing to pain. Sedated and currently on propofol.

What blood test(s) will you order?

CBC	WBC	16 x $10^3/\mu L$
	Hemoglobin	9g/dL
	Hematocrit	28%
	Platelets	550 x $10^3/\mu L$
CHEM-6	Na	134mEq/L
	K	5.2mEq/L
	Cl	95mEq/L
	Bicarbonate	11mEq/L
	BUN	20mg/dL
	Creatinine	1.6mg/dL
LFTS	AST	1950 units/L
	ALT	2500 units/L
	Alkaline phosphatase	190 units/L
	Total bilirubin	2.5mg/dL
INR		1.0
Lactate		5.2mmol/L

Does this change your differential diagnosis?

Yes. The patient's laboratory data demonstrate sequelae of systemic hypoperfusion evidenced by acute kidney injury, an elevated lactate level, high anion gap metabolic acidosis, and likely ischemic hepatitis. Given this, the likely diagnosis for the lower GI bleed is acute ischemic colitis.

How will you proceed?

The patient clearly has chronic systolic dysfunction, and probably had an acute decompensation and/or a septic event leading to shock (i.e., cardiogenic vs. septic shock). Either way, her colonic mucosa was perturbed by acute hypoperfusion and resultant vasoconstriction to divert blood to other vital organs. In this delicate clinical state, an urgent sigmoidoscopy may not reveal anything to change the patient's overall management.

A more conservative approach might involve simply improving her hemodynamics and treating the underlying condition. Given this, a CT scan is performed to evaluate the extent of ischemia (Figures 89 and 90).

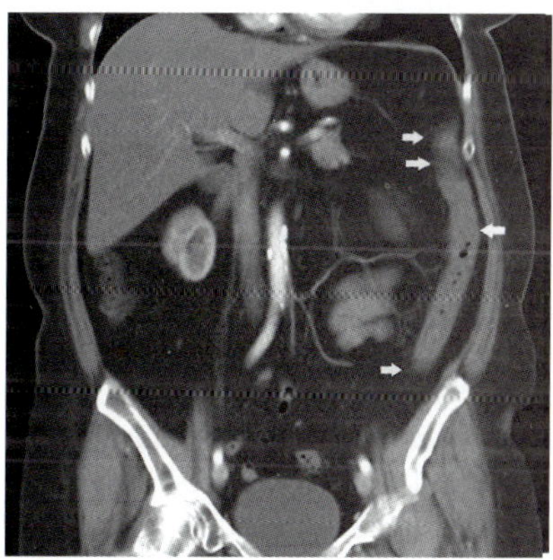

Figure 89. *Image Coutesy of Dr. Dmitry Rakita.*

Describe what you see and read on

The coronal image of the abdomen with IV contrast (Figure 89) shows mild circumferential wall thickening of the descending colon (white arrow). There is minimal pericolonic inflammation (yellow arrows) with no evidence of pneumatosis or pneumoperitoneum.

The sagittal image (Figure 90) demonstrates a moderate degree of atherosclerotic calcification at the origins of the celiac artery and superior mesenteric artery off of the aorta (black arrows). A small fat-containing umbilical hernia is incidentally noted (white star).

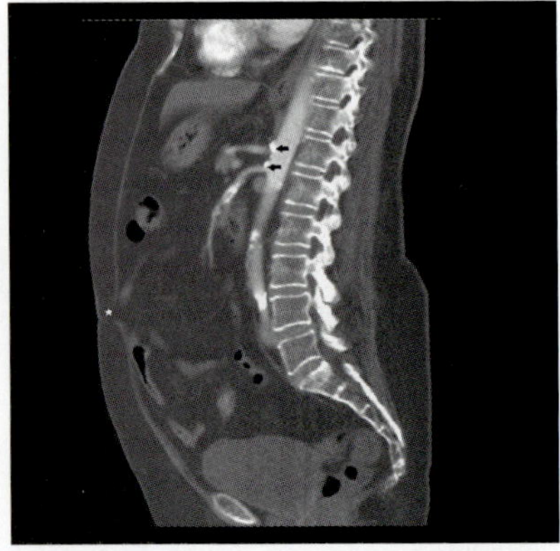

Figure 90. *Image Coutesy of Dr. Dmitry Rakita.*

Clinical pearls

- Ischemic colitis is usually a result of either acute or chronic mesenteric ischemia. In some patients, pre-existing atherosclerotic disease of the mesenteric vessels can predispose to an acute-on-chronic injury.
- Systemic hypoperfusion and splanchnic vasoconstriction lead to bowel damage, resulting in bowel wall distension and fluid/protein leakage. In addition, this can lead to bacterial translocation and, therefore, systemic bacteremia.
- In mild cases the initial treatment is usually supportive, with IV fluids, serial abdominal examinations, and close follow-up of laboratory values.

Impress your attending

What are the typical endoscopic findings with ischemic colitis?

Bowel wall necrosis, friability, ulceration, edema, and pale mucosa.

Apart from supportive care and fluids, what else may be given for moderate to severe cases of ischemic colitis in this scenario?

Parenteral antibiotics are reasonable given the likelihood of bacterial translocation and secondary infectious complications from severe colitis.

Case 41

A 35-year-old woman presents to the hepatology clinic for evaluation of a small echogenic mass found on an abdominal ultrasound performed in the office of her primary-care physician. The patient initially presented to her primary-care physician a month ago for abdominal pain, which has now resolved. At the time the pain was located in the right upper quadrant. It was a dull, achy pain that was non-radiating. There were no exacerbating or alleviating factors.

The patient denies nausea, vomiting, or change in her bowel habits. Moreover, she has not had fevers, chills, or weight loss. She does not have other GI symptoms, and has no significant past medical history. She has never had abdominal surgery or received a blood transfusion. She currently lives with her boyfriend and has been taking oral contraceptives for the past 10 years. She is not on any other medications. She has not recently traveled to a foreign destination. There is no history of IV drug use. She drinks alcohol socially and is a non-smoker.

Physical examination

Vitals	Temperature 97.9°F, HR 55 bpm, BP 115/80mmHg, oxygen saturation 100% on RA.
GEN	No obvious distress.
HEENT	Moist mucous membranes. No scleral icterus. No lymphadenopathy.
CVS	Normal S1, S2. No murmurs, rubs, or gallops.
RESP	Clear to auscultation.
ABD	Soft and non-tender. No appreciable ascites or palpable splenomegaly. Rectal examination deferred.
EXT	No clubbing, cyanosis, or edema.

What blood test(s) will you order?

CBC	WBC	7.5 x 103/µL
	Hemoglobin	14g/dL
	Hematocrit	42%
	Platelets	350 x 10^3/µL
CHEM	Na	138mEq/L
	K	4.9mEq/L
	Creatinine	0.7mEq/L
LFTs	AST	25 units/L
	ALT	30 units/L
	Alkaline phosphatase	140 units/L
	Total bilirubin	0.8mg/dL
INR		0.9

The α-fetoprotein level is within normal limits.

How will you proceed?

The clinical presentation is of a young, healthy woman with an incidental

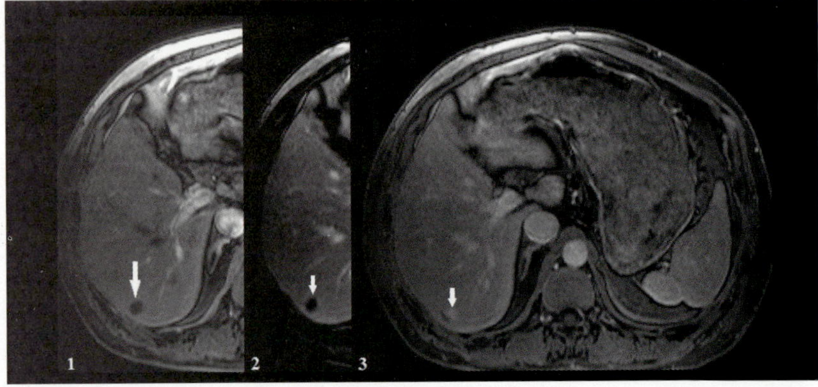

Figure 91. *Image Coutesy of Dr. Dmitry Rakita.*

finding of an abdominal mass. She no longer has abdominal pain and has a benign abdominal examination. She does not appear clinically to have cirrhosis.

What imaging test will you order?

Although a CT scan of the liver may prove diagnostic, MRI may be a more appropriate choice given the lack of ionizing radiation. The resulting images are shown in Figure 91.

Describe what you see and read on

An MRI was performed in multiple sequences:

- 1. hepatic-arterial;
- 2. portal venous; and
- 3. equilibrium.

Imaging demonstrates a 1.5cm lesion in the posterior segment of the right hepatic lobe. The lesion (white arrows) demonstrates peripheral nodular enhancement in the hepatic-arterial phase. This is followed by progressive centripetal filling during the portal venous phase, and subsequently hyperintensity (relative to the liver) during the equilibrium phase.

What is the most likely cause and what else should be ruled out?

The MRI shows the typical features of a liver hemangioma. Checking the α-fetoprotein level was prudent. The combination of a normal α-fetoprotein level, no risk factors for hepatocellular carcinoma, and the typical enhancing pattern of a hemangioma supports this likely diagnosis.

Given the size of the lesion, how will you manage the hemangioma?

Treatment is rarely required unless the patient exhibits symptoms (i.e., rupture, pain, localized compression symptoms, platelet sequestration), in which case arterial embolization or surgical resection can be performed. If the patient is asymptomatic and the lesion is less than 1.5cm in size, the patient can often be reassured and observed.

Clinical pearls

- Hemangiomas are a common incidental finding on imaging performed for the evaluation of abdominal pain of other etiologies. It is interesting that this patient's pain resolved by the time she saw a hepatologist, and it is likely her pain was caused by an entirely different phenomenon such as reflux or non-ulcer dyspepsia.

- Hemangiomas are the most common benign liver lesions. They are most common in women in their 20s and 30s.
- The risks of using oral contraceptives are not well understood. The link of estrogen to hemangioma size is controversial. Moreover, oral contraceptives have an association with hepatic adenomas.
- MRI easily distinguishes hemangiomas from hepatocellular carcinoma.
- Biopsies are not necessary to diagnose hemangiomas.

Impress your attending

If the MRI was inconclusive in determining the lesion type, what other imaging studies might you have obtained?

- Three-phase CT scan of the liver.
- Technetium-99m-pertechnetate RBC pool study.

Case 42

A 28-year-old woman is admitted from her primary-care physician's office with intractable nausea and vomiting for the past few months. She vomits several times daily and has difficulty keeping food down. The vomiting usually occurs shortly after meals, and generally consists of food contents. She denies abdominal pain, changes in bowel habit, hematochezia, or melena. Her stools have been normal in consistency. She occasionally feels bloated after meals.

The patient has no history of GI disease. Her past medical history is significant for longstanding type 1 diabetes mellitus since childhood. She appears to have poor control of her diabetes, as evidenced by her most recent HbA1c value of 9.5%. In addition to her insulin regimen, she was recently started on paroxetine for mild depression. She lives with her boyfriend. She occasionally drinks alcohol and is a non-smoker. The family history is negative for gastric or esophageal neoplasia; her mother had a cholecystectomy.

What is your differential diagnosis?

The differential diagnosis includes gastroenteritis, medication side effect,gastroparesis, gastroesophageal reflux disease, cholecystitis/ symptomatic cholelithiasis, and (less likely) mechanical obstruction.

Physical examination

Vitals Temperature 99.0°F, HR 99 bpm, BP 110/75mmHg, oxygen saturation 98% on RA.

GEN Appears tired.

HEENT Dry mucous membranes. No scleral icterus. No lymphadenopathy.

CVS Normal S1, S2. No murmurs, rubs, or gallops.

RESP Clear to auscultation.

ABD Soft and non-tender. No succussion splash. Bowels sounds are normal.

EXT No edema.

What blood test(s) will you order?

CBC	WBC	8.5 x 10^3/μL
	Hemoglobin	14.2g/dL
	Hematocrit	42%
	Platelets	400 x 10^3/μL
CHEM-6	Na	136mEq/L
	K	4.6mEq/L
	Cl	110mEq/L
	Bicarbonate	24mEq/L
	Creatinine	0.8mg/dL
	Glucose	330mg/dL
LFTs	AST	23 units/L
	ALT	30 units/L
	Alkaline phosphatase	25 units/L
	Total bilirubin	0.7mg/dL

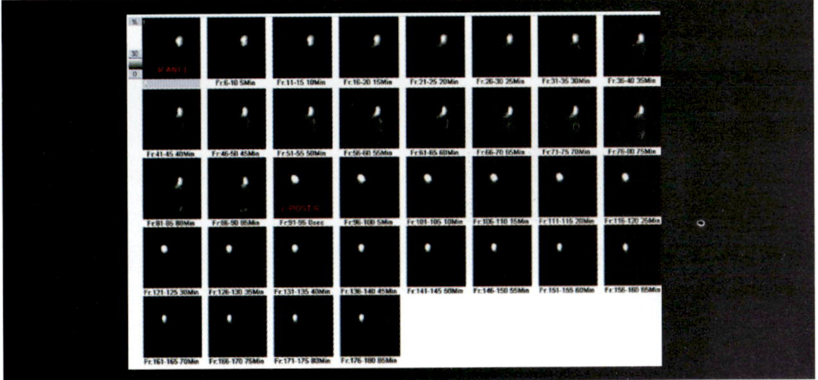

Figure 92.

How will you proceed?

Given the normal bowel sounds, and that the patient is having normal bowel movements, both obstruction and ileus are less likely. The patient undergoes an abdominal radiograph that confirms a normal bowel gas pattern.

The patient appears mildly dehydrated clinically. In addition, she has hyperglycemia from poorly controlled type 1 diabetes mellitus. She does not have ketoacidosis, but she continues to vomit any ingested food, even liquids. The patient should be initially placed on IV fluids and an insulin regimen to control her blood glucose.

The next day the patient is feeling better. However, after breakfast she still complains of early satiety, nausea, vomiting, and postprandial abdominal fullness. Given the patient has a longstanding history of uncontrolled diabetes, gastroparesis is the likely diagnosis.

The next step is to order a nuclear gastric-emptying study (scintigraphy) (Figures 92 and 93).

A solid-phase, 90-minute gastric-emptying study is performed. The patient is given 1mCi of Tc99m sulfur colloid in a fried egg-white toast sandwich with 7oz of water. Dynamic anterior and posterior views of the abdomen are acquired and the percentage emptying at 90 minutes is calculated using a geometric mean.

Dynamic images demonstrate no esophageal activity during the examination to suggest poor esophageal transit or reflux. Gastric contour is normal. There is a lag phase of approximately 20 minutes, followed by gradual diminished emptying from the stomach into the small bowel. The percentage of gastric emptying at 90 minutes is calculated to be 22%.

Solid gastric emptying of less than 34% at 90 minutes is considered abnormal. Therefore, the impression of this study is that there is delayed gastric emptying.

How will you treat the patient?

Optimizing the patient's glycemic control is the first priority. A trial of 10mg of metoclopramide 30 minutes prior to meals should be given.

Given the patient's young age and her diabetes, which is an obvious risk factor for gastroparesis, mechanical obstruction (as from gastric malignancy) is not suspected. Therefore, endoscopy is not needed unless the patient has refractory symptoms.

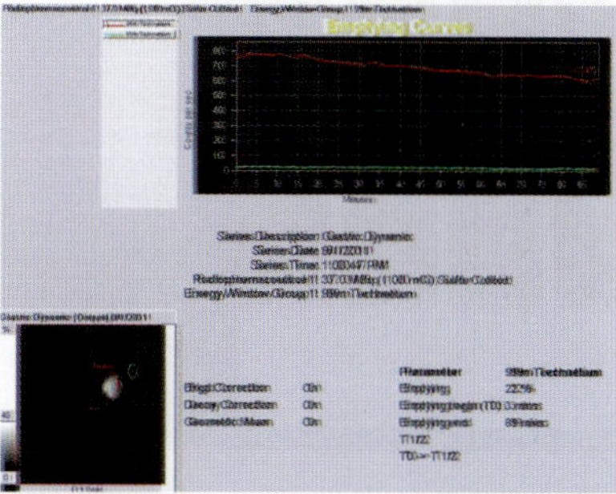

Figure 93.

Clinical pearls

- Gastroparesis is part of an autonomic neuropathy that can present with various manifestations, including bloating, early satiety, postprandial nausea and vomiting, and abdominal pain.
- Gastroparesis may be found in patients with diabetic autonomic neuropathy.

Impress your attending

How would you prepare a patient for scintigraphy?

Scintigraphy is usually performed after an overnight fast. In addition, drugs that accelerate or delay gastric emptying must be temporarily stopped.

Case 43

A 50-year-old man presents with 3 days of nausea and vomiting. He also has a constant abdominal pain in the right upper quadrant. He has lost his appetite, and has recently noticed tea-colored urine and yellowing of his eyes. He feels he has a low-grade fever but no chills. He has not lost weight.

The patient's past medical history is significant for hypertension, obesity, and hypothyroidism. He has not undergone surgery in the past. He lives at home with his wife and children. He does not smoke cigarettes or drink alcohol. None of his contacts are unwell, he has not traveled recently, and he has no tattoos.

Physical examination

Vitals	Temperature 101.10F, HR 110 bpm, BP 130/90mmHg, oxygen saturation 97% on RA.
GEN	In obvious distress.
HEENT	Icterus. Neck supple and no jugular venous distension.
CVS	Normal S1, S2. No murmurs, rubs, or gallops.
RESP	Clear to auscultation bilaterally.
ABD	Right upper quadrant tenderness with a negative Murphy's sign. No guarding. Bowel sounds are normal.
EXT	No edema.
Skin	No spider nevi or palmar erythema.

What blood test(s) will you order?

CBC	**WBC**	16 x $10^3/\mu L$
	Hemoglobin	13.5g/dL
	Hematocrit	40%
	Platelets	500 x $10^3/\mu L$
CHEM-7		Within normal limits
LFTs	**AST**	40 units/L
	ALT	50 units/L
	Alkaline phosphatase	460 units/L
	Total bilirubin	3.2mg/dL
Lipase		45 units/L

What is the differential diagnosis, and how will you proceed?

This is a patient with right upper quadrant pain, fever, and jaundice, fulfilling Charcot's triad of cholangitis. The causes of cholangitis include choledocholithiasis, Mirizzi syndrome, primary sclerosing cholangitis, secondary sclerosing cholangitis, pancreatic mass, and biliary malignancy. The patient undergoes an abdominal ultrasound for initial imaging, which reveals a normal-sized common bile duct.

What imaging test will you order?

Given the differential diagnosis, the next step is either a CT scan of the abdomen (to look for a mass or signs of biliary obstruction) or an MRCP for better visualization of biliary strictures. An MRCP is obtained in this patient (Figure 94).

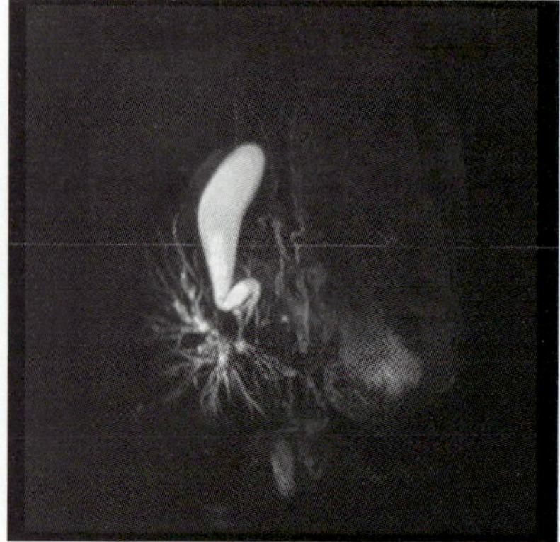

Figure 94.

Describe what you see and read on

A coronal maximum-intensity projection MRCP is shown. There is moderate to severe intrahepatic biliary ductal dilatation. Strictures are present involving the distal right and left lobar branches, as well as distal segmental strictures. Filling defects are seen predominantly in the right lobe, probably representing debris. The extrahepatic biliary tree is not dilated. The cystic duct and gallbladder are unremarkable. The common hepatic duct just below the hilum is slightly irregular and becomes larger in caliber at its mid-portion. The gallbladder is normally distended and unremarkable, without evidence of cholelithiasis. These findings were not noted on ultrasound, which does not have sufficient sensitivity to delineate these abnormalities.

Given the radiology findings, how will you manage this patient?

This patient has biliary strictures without stone disease; he may have primary sclerosing cholangitis. Secondary causes such as HIV should be ruled out. Primary sclerosing cholangitis is associated with positive autoimmune markers (ANA, p-ANCA). Given the patient's initial presentation, blood cultures should be drawn and parenteral antibiotics (Gram-negative coverage) started and continued for at least 1 week.

Although the MRCP did not show any dominant strictures, these should be ruled out with ERCP. If a dominant stricture is found at ERCP, it can be dilated and stented at that time. In addition, dominant strictures pose a risk of malignancy, so brushings for cytology and endoscopic biopsies can be obtained if a stricture is present. Figure 95 shows an ERCP image from a different patient with primary sclerosing cholangitis, who has a similar hilar stricture (white arrow), that ultimately required dilatation and stenting.

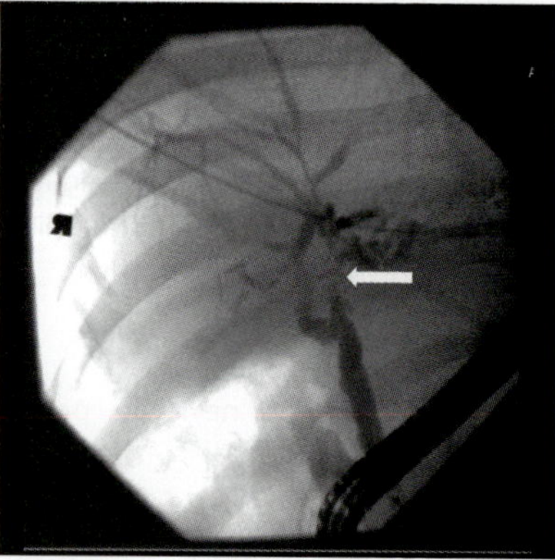

Figure 95.

Note that the above patient in Figure 95 has had a prior cholecystectomy, and there are clips on the cystic duct remnant and cystic artery. The intrahepatic ducts show characteristic pruning and segmental stricturing. Endoscopic management of dominant strictures may lead to improved long-term outcomes. There are no data to support long-term prophylactic antibiotic use in patients with primary sclerosing cholangitis, but most physicians would advocate temporary antibiotic coverage after elective endoscopic management (ERCP).

Clinical pearls

- Primary sclerosing cholangitis is a risk factor for cholangiocarcinoma, and surveillance with serum CA 19.9 and imaging (i.e., MRI) should be performed annually.
- Primary sclerosing cholangitis shows characteristic multifocal stricturing of intrahepatic and/or extrahepatic bile ducts.
- An exacerbation (infection) should be treated with antibiotics.
- Chronic therapy involves ursodeoxycholic acid. However, this has not been shown to improve morbidity or mortality. Cholestyramine, a bile acid sequestrant, is also given for pruritus.

Impress your attending

What must be performed if the patient has evidence of a dominant stricture?

The patient should have an ERCP, with dilatation or stenting if potentially required.

What additional cancers are associated with primary sclerosing cholangitis?

Colon cancer, gallbladder cancer, and cholangiocarcinoma.

What does the patient need if ERCP fails or is technically difficult?

The patient may need percutaneous transhepatic cholangiography with biliary drainage by interventional radiology.

What is the definitive treatment of primary sclerosing cholangitis?

Liver transplantation.

Case 44

A 50-year-old woman is referred to the gastroenterology clinic from her primary-care physician. She presented to her primary-care physician a week ago with at least 2-3 months of generalized weakness. She cannot pinpoint when the fatigue began. She has found herself falling asleep at work, and no longer has the energy to carry out normal daily activities. Other than this profound fatigue she denies symptoms of hypothyroidism or depression, and has not been started on any new medications. Over the past week or so she has developed terrible itching, which has kept her up at night. Her husband has noticed yellowing of her skin.

The patient denies abdominal pain, nausea, vomiting, or changes in the consistency or appearance of her bowel motions. Her weight has been stable. She rarely drinks alcohol. Her past medical history is significant for hypothyroidism, and she is currently taking levothyroxine. The patient is a homemaker. She has not traveled recently and none of her contacts are unwell. She has three children, for which all pregnancies were uncomplicated.

Physical examination

Vitals Temperature 98.5°F, HR 60 bpm, BP 130/70mmHg, oxygen saturation 99% on RA.

GEN No distress. No fetor hepaticus.

HEENT Jaundiced and icteric. Moist mucous membranes.

CVS Normal S1, S2. No murmurs, rubs, or gallops.

RESP Clear to auscultation bilaterally.

ABD Soft and non-tender. One or more fingerbreadth non-tender hepatomegaly. No splenomegaly. No appreciable ascites. Bowel sounds are normal.

Skin Warm. No needle-track marks or extremity edema. No tattoos, spider nevi, or palmar erythema.

NEURO Alert and orientated to time, place, and person. No asterixis.

What blood test(s) will you order?

CBC	WBC	8.5 x 10^3/μL
	Hemoglobin	13.0g/dL
	Hematocrit	39%
	Platelets	390 x 10^3/μL
CHEM-6	Na	135mEq/L
	K	4.2mEq/L
	Cl	110mEq/L
	Bicarbonate	26mEq/L
	BUN	15mg/dL
	Creatinine	0.9mg/dL
LFTs	AST	60 units/L
	ALT	50 units/L
	Alkaline phosphatase	350 units/L

Total bilirubin	4.5mg/dL
GGT	120 units/L

What imaging test will you order?

An ultrasound of the right upper quadrant is obtained (Figure 96).

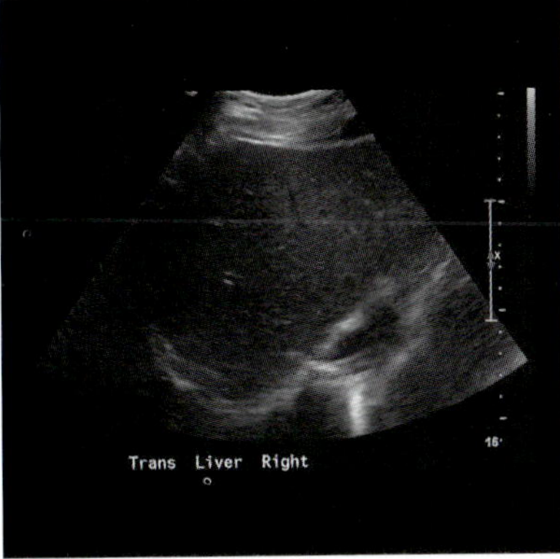

Figure 96.

Describe what you see and read on

A transverse grayscale image of the liver is shown. The liver is of normal echogenicity and texture, but is slightly enlarged. There are no focal hepatic lesions. Although not shown, the common bile duct is of normal caliber without evidence of obstruction, and the spleen and gallbladder are normal.

What is your differential diagnosis?

This patient's main presentation was fatigue, jaundice, and pruritus. Her LFTs suggest an obstructive process, but her biliary tree is normal in appearance. This essentially rules out gallstone pathology. An obstructive pattern of LFTs, characterized by elevated alkaline phosphatase and GGT levels, suggests possible intrahepatic biliary obstruction. The patient's past medical history of hypothyroidism — an autoimmune disease — places primary biliary cirrhosis at the top of the differential diagnosis list.

Given the history of autoimmune disease, what is the next step in the work-up?

Autoimmune testing should be performed next, including AMA, serum IgG, and anti-smooth muscle antibody.

The results are as follows:

AMA	Positive titer of 1:250
Serum IgG	3500mg/dL (normal <1600mg/dL)
Anti-smooth muscle antibody	Negative

The patient undergoes a liver biopsy. This demonstrates the typical features of primary biliary cirrhosis, with portal hepatitis and granuloma. There is no evidence of fibrosis. The patient should be started on ursodeoxycholic acid (10-15mg/kg/day orally), and cholestyramine (4g four times a day orally) for pruritus. She should be scheduled for a DEXA scan to screen for osteoporosis and osteopenia.

Clinical pearls

- Liver biopsy is not always required for a diagnosis of primary biliary cirrhosis if typical features, including a positive AMA result, are present (95% of cases). Biopsy is sometimes needed for prognostic or staging reasons.
- Biopsy (and other serologic testing) may be needed to rule out autoimmune hepatitis, since an overlap syndrome can exist between the two diseases. Autoimmune hepatitis usually results in higher

levels of AST and ALT (potentially in the thousands).

- Up to a third of patients with primary biliary cirrhosis experience osteoporosis and osteopenia. The severity of these is often correlated with the severity of the primary biliary cirrhosis. Screening with a DEXA scan is recommended.

Impress your attending

What other intrahepatic cholestatic diseases are there?

Other intrahepatic cholestatic diseases include drug-induced cholestasis, primary sclerosing cholangitis, Caroli's disease, intrahepatic cholestasis of pregnancy, and progressive familial intrahepatic cholestasis. Infiltrating diseases such as sarcoidosis, amyloidosis, and infiltrating neoplasms can also give a cholestatic picture.

Case 45

A 65-year-old man presents to his primary-care physician with painless jaundice. He denies nausea or vomiting. His stools have not changed in appearance, but he has noticed dark-colored urine. He has had an unintended weight loss of more than 15 lbs in the past 2 months.

The patient has not experienced fevers or chills. He does not have risk factors for viral hepatitis such as a blood transfusion, tattoos, or IV drug use. He is a chronic cigarette smoker (one pack per day) for more than 40 years and drinks at least one alcoholic drink daily. There is no family history of GI disease. The patient's past medical history is significant for hypertension, for which he takes hydrochlorothiazide. He does not take any other prescription medications, over-the-counter medications, or herbal supplements, and has no reported allergies.

What is your differential diagnosis?

The differential diagnosis includes choledocholithiasis, alcoholic hepatitis, other toxic ingestion, cholangiocarcinoma or gallbladder carcinoma, pancreatic cancer, metastatic cancer, and bile duct strictures.

Physical examination

Vitals	Temperature 98.5°F, HR 75 bpm, BP 120/75mmHg, oxygen saturation 99% on RA.
GEN	Jaundice. No obvious distress.
HEENT	Scleral icterus and moist mucous membranes. No lymphadenopathy.
CVS	Normal S1, S2. No murmurs, rubs, or gallops.
RESP	Clear to auscultation.
ABD	Obese. Soft and non-tender. No appreciable ascites. Bowel sounds are normal.
EXT	No clubbing or edema.

Do these findings change your differential diagnosis?

No. The physical examination findings can still point to any diagnosis. If the patient had a palpable gallbladder, this would suggest the presence of distal bile duct obstruction as from a pancreatic head mass; this is called Courvoisier's sign.

What blood test(s) will you order?

CBC	WBC	11.5 x 10^3/μL
	Hemoglobin	12g/dL
	Hematocrit	36%
	Platelets	315 x 10^3/μL
CHEM-7	Na	138mEq/L
	K	3.8mEq/L
	Cl	104mEq/L
	Bicarbonate	26mEq/L
	BUN	13mg/dL
	Creatinine	0.8mg/dL
	Glucose	110mg/dL
LFTs	AST	104 units/L

	ALT	59 units/L
	Alkaline phosphatase	279 units/L
	Total bilirubin (direct 13.8mg/dL)	19.7mg/dL
INR		1.2

How would you interpret the abnormal LFTs?

Given the markedly elevated bilirubin and alkaline phosphatase levels, the pattern of abnormalities is suggestive of a cholestatic process. However, the transaminases are also elevated — specifically the AST/ALT ratio. This can be seen with alcoholic hepatitis. Severe alcoholic hepatitis can also result in cholestasis and an elevated bilirubin level.

What imaging test will you order?

The patient undergoes a CT scan of the abdomen (Figure 97).

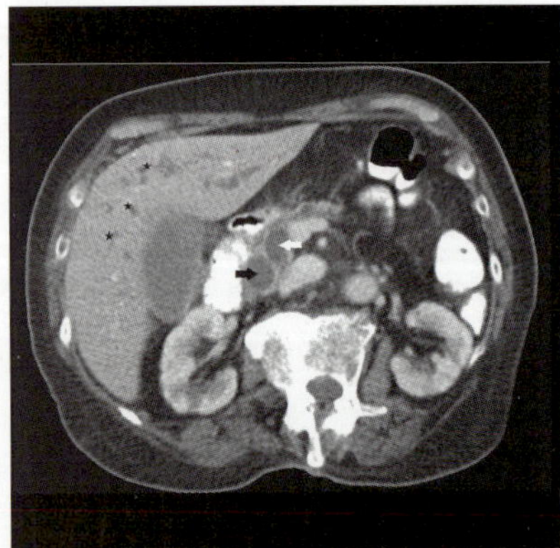

Figure 97.

Describe what you see and read on

Figure 97 shows a single axial image of the abdomen with IV and oral contrast. There is massive dilatation of the common bile duct (black arrow) and pancreatic duct (white arrow). Intrahepatic biliary ducts are also noted to be dilated (black stars). Although not shown on this image, more inferiorly there was an ill-defined mass at the pancreatic head or uncinate process. There was no definite evidence of vascular encasement or invasion of the portal vein, superior mesenteric vein, or superior mesenteric artery.

Given the obstructive process is probably being caused by a pancreatic mass, the patient should be referred for an ERCP for stent placement to clear his jaundice and to obtain brush cytology and forceps biopsies. Alternatively, an endoscopic ultrasound with fine-needle aspiration could be performed; however, the patient would remain jaundiced.

Some surgeons advocate taking a jaundiced patient such as this directly for a Whipple procedure without stenting, because retrospective, non-randomized data suggest a lower infection rate without preoperative stenting. However, most surgeons would prefer a preoperative tissue diagnosis, especially in this patient, who has a long history of smoking and a reversed transaminase ratio suggestive of considerable alcohol use.

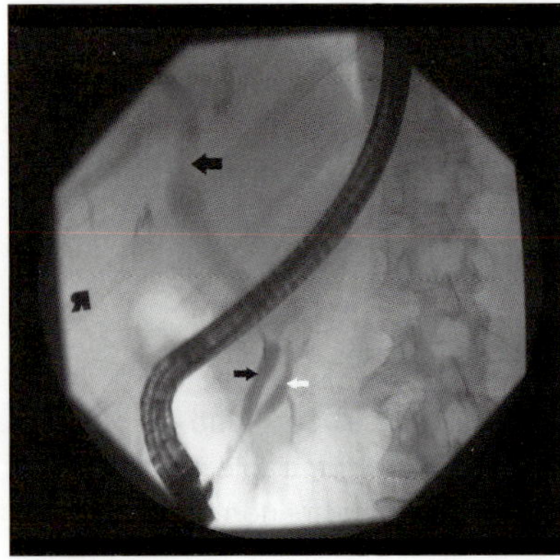

Figure 98.

Describe what you see and read on

Figure 98 shows a single fluoroscopic image from a similar patient obtained during an ERCP, demonstrating a cannulated common bile duct. Contrast injection reveals that both the common bile duct (small black arrow) and pancreatic duct (white arrow) are dilated, with abrupt narrowing or stricturing at the level of a mass. Note the dilated common hepatic duct (large black arrow) above the stricture.

The patient underwent biliary sphincterotomy, forceps and brush biopsies of the strictured area, and placement of a plastic biliary stent. Brush cytology returned a diagnosis of adenocarcinoma of the pancreas.

Given the diagnosis, how will you proceed?

The patient should be evaluated by a surgical team for the possibility of tumor resection. In the interim, the biliary stent will temporarily relieve the obstruction.

Clinical pearls

- Pancreatic cancer, specifically in the pancreatichead, can present with painless jaundice.
- Biliary obstruction causes cholestasis, resulting in elevated transaminase, bilirubin, and alkaline phosphatase levels.
- Stenting is a temporary measure in surgical candidates, and is otherwise palliative in non-surgical candidates.

Impress your attending

What is the surgical treatment for cancer of the pancreatic head?

Curative management is by means of a Whipple procedure (i.e., resection of the pancreatic head and duodenum, with gastrojejunostomy, pancreatico-jejunostomy, and choledochojejunostomy). A subtotal pancreatectomy is the treatment of choice for cancer of the tail and body of the pancreas.

Case 46

A 42-year-old man is referred to the gastroenterology clinic for work-up of abnormal LFTs. As part of routine testing by his primary-care physician, he was found to have an AST level of 50 units/L and an ALT level of 70 units/L. His alkaline phosphatase and total bilirubin levels were within normal limits.

The patient's past medical history is significant for type 2 diabetes, hypertension, and dyslipidemia. He was started on metformin 4 months ago for newly detected diabetes, and his other medication doses (of hydrochlorothiazide and simvastatin) have remained the same. He rarely drinks alcohol, has not traveled abroad, and has never used IV drugs. He does not take over-the-counter medications or herbal supplements. As part of the patient's work-up, his primary-care physician ordered an abdominal ultrasound (Figure 99).

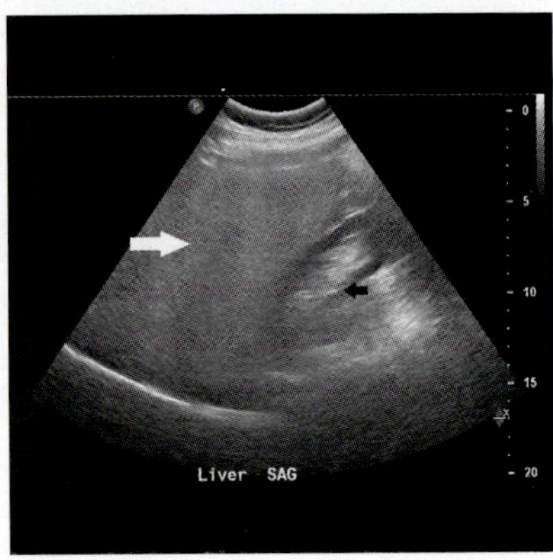

Figure 99.

Describe what you see and read on

This single sagittal image shows an echogenic liver (white arrow). There is normal echotexture and no focal hepatic abnormality. There is no evidence of perihepatic fluid. Other images (not shown) show the liver has a normal surface contour. The black arrow shows the right kidney.

Physical examination

Vitals	Temperature 97.4°F, HR 60 bpm, BP 120/86mmHg, oxygen saturation 99% on RA.
GEN	No obvious distress.
HEENT	Moist mucous membranes. No scleral icterus. No lymphadenopathy.
CVS	Normal S1, S2. No murmurs, rubs, or gallops.
RESP	Clear to auscultation.
ABD	Soft and non-tender. No hepato¬splenomegaly. Normal bowel sounds.
EXT	No clubbing or edema.

What blood test(s) will you order?

CBC	WBC	6.5 x 10^3/μL
	Hemoglobin	15.2g/dL
	Hematocrit	45%

	Platelets	380 x 10^3/µL
CHEM-6	Na	139mEq/L
	K	3.9mEq/L
	Cl	119mEq/L
	Bicarbonate	25mEq/L
	BUN	10mg/dL
	Creatinine	0.9mg/dL
INR		0.9

A decision is made to undertake further evaluation of the echogenic liver, as the differential diagnosis for this includes hepatic steatosis, hepatitis, and in some cases cirrhosis.

What other laboratory tests will you order?

- Hepatitis C antibody.
- Hepatitis B surface antigen.
- Hepatitis B surface antibody.
- AMA.
- ANA.
- Anti-smooth muscle antibody.
- Serum IgG.
- Ceruloplasmin.
- α-1 anti-trypsin.
- IFerritin.
- Iron.
- Total iron-binding capacity.

All of the above tests return as negative or within normal limits.

Other blood tests return and show the following

HbA1c is elevated at 8.5%.

Insulin is elevated at 18µIU/mL, and the fasting glucose level measures 160mg/dL.

What is the most likely diagnosis, and how will you proceed?

The patient most probably has non-alcoholic fatty liver disease. The pattern of LIFT abnormalities (elevated AST and ALT levels, with an AST/ALT ratio <1) and the patient's risk factor of the metabolic syndrome is highly suggestive of this. Importantly, other causes of liver disease have been excluded. In addition, the patient has poorly controlled diabetes and evidence of insulin resistance (based on the insulin to glucose ratio).

What else might you consider doing?

A definitive diagnosis of non-alcoholic fatty liver disease requires a liver biopsy, which will show the typical features of steatosis. Some patients, however, have inflammation, which indicates a condition known as non-alcoholic steatohepatitis. These patients have a more aggressive form of fatty liver disease that can lead to cirrhosis. Risk factors for non-alcoholic steatohepatitis include age older than 45 years, body-mass index higher than 30kg/m2, type 2 diabetes mellitus, and an AST to ALT ratio higher than 1.

A conservative approach to non-alcoholic fatty liver disease is to prescribe lifestyle changes and tight control of comorbidities such as diabetes, and follow LIFT improvements before performing a liver biopsy. Histological staging for non-alcoholic steatohepatitis depends on the presence and degree of inflammation, ballooning, and steatosis.

Clinical pearls

- Non-alcoholic fatty liver disease is often asymptomatic. Non-alcoholic steatohepatitis is a more aggressive form characterized by inflammation that may lead to cirrhosis.

- The presence of an echogenic liver may be inferred by comparing the liver parenchyma to the renal cortex, and being unable to distinguish the portal triad in the liver parenchyma.

Impress your attending

What makes up the metabolic syndrome?

Based on the National Cholesterol Education Program — Adult Treatment Panel, three of five criteria must be met:

- Waist circumference of more than 40 inches for men and 35 inches for women.
- A triglyceride level of 150mg/dL or higher or
- current treatment for elevated triglycerides. High-density lipoprotein cholesterol of less than 40mg/dL for men or 50mg/dL for women.
- Hypertension, with a blood pressure of 130/85mmHg or higher.
- A fasting blood glucose level of 100mg/dL or higher.

Case 47

A 65-year-old woman is admitted with a 2-day history of worsening abdominal pain. She describes the pain as cramping in nature. It is generalized and does not radiate. The patient has repeatedly vomited in the past 24 hours, but did not notice blood in her vomit. Her last bowel movement was 3 days ago and was normal in consistency. She has suffered from constipation and hard stools in the past. She has not passed flatus in the past day. She denies melena or hematochezia.

The patient's past medical history is significant for coronary artery disease, type 2 diabetes mellitus, and chronic atrial fibrillation. She has had multiple abdominal surgeries, including an emergency appendectomy and a hysterectomy for fibroids. Her medications include metoprolol, lisinopril, warfarin, simvastatin, and metformin. She lives at home with her husband and stopped smoking 20 years ago. She rarely drinks alcohol.

What is your differential diagnosis?

The differential diagnosis includes constipation, small-bowel obstruction, large-bowel obstruction, diverticulitis, mesenteric ischemia, and possibly pancreatitis.

Physical examination

Vitals	Temperature 99.0°F, HR 90 bpm, BP 145/85mmHg, oxygen saturation 96% on RA.
GEN	Mild general distress.
HEENT	Dry mucous membranes. No scleral icterus. No lymphadenopathy.
CVS	Irregularly irregular rhythm. No murmurs, rubs, or gallops.
RESP	Clear to auscultation.
ABD	Distended abdomen, tympanic to percussion throughout. Bowel sounds are hyperactive. Empty rectal vault on examination without blood on the glove.
EXT	No clubbing or edema.

What blood test(s) will you order?

CBC	**WBC**	17.2 x 10^3/μL
	Hemoglobin	12.1g/dL
	HCT	39.8%
	Platelets	520 x 10^3/μL
CHEM	**Na**	134mEq/L
	K	4.8mEq/L
	Cl	112mEq/L
	Bicarbonate	17mEq/L
	Creatinine	1.1mEq/L
LFTs	**AST**	30 units/L
	ALT	35 units/L
	Alkaline phosphatase	111 units/L

Total bilirubin	0.8mg/dL
INR	2.0
Lactate	2.1mmol/L
Lipase	526 units/L

What imaging test will you order?

A plain film of the abdomen is ordered (Figure 100).

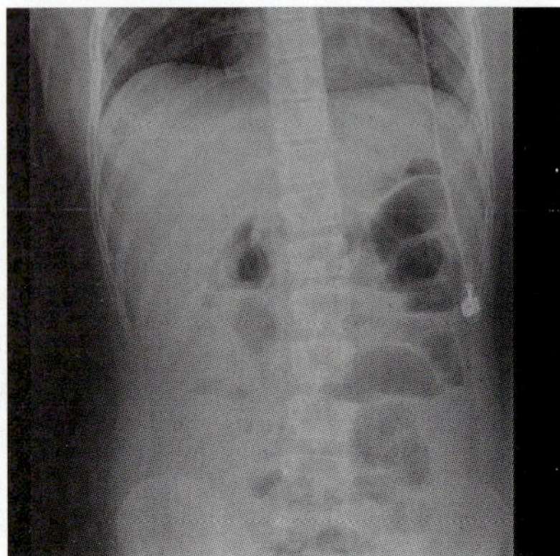

Figure 100.

Describe what you see and read on

This upright plain film of the abdomen demonstrates at least three air-fluid levels on the left. No gas is seen in the colon. Soft-tissue outlines are unremarkable. There are no abnormal calcifications or acute osseous abnormalities. These findings are concerning for a small-bowel obstruction centered in the mid-abdomen.

How will you proceed?

The patient has evidence of an acute small-bowel obstruction. The immediate management involves resuscitation and bowel rest. The patient should be admitted to the surgical service, placed on nasogastric suction, and started on IV fluids. She should also undergo serial abdominal examinations. Her warfarin should be stopped and she should be put on low-molecular-weight heparin.

The patient fails to improve over the next day; instead, her pain and distension worsen. Her BP begins to fall and she becomes tachycardic. She is taken for an explorative laparotomy for small-bowel obstruction. She is found to have adhesions in the mid-jejunum, which are treated with lysis. The patient's bowel demonstrates good color, and her mesenteric vessels are pulsatile and normal in appearance. She recovers well after surgery.

Clinical pearls

- Most small-bowel obstruction cases are caused by adhesions and hernias.
- Patients on warfarin who will potentially require urgent surgery should be switched to anticoagulation with heparin because of its shorter half-life.
- Mesenteric ischemia is an important differential diagnosis in any patient with vascular disease or atrial fibrillation.
- Abdominal CT scans can further characterize bowel obstructions, often giving the exact transition point. In this case, the patient became unstable and the CT scan was bypassed.

Impress your attending

What other causes of small-bowel obstruction can you name?

Causes of small-bowel obstruction include adhesions, malignancy, hernias, strictures, early postoperative obstruction, trauma, intussusception, bezoars, gallstone ileus, and superior mesenteric artery syndrome.

Why was this patient's lipase elevated?

Small-bowel obstruction (and also ileus, acute mesenteric ischemia, active small-bowel Crohn's disease, and peptic ulcer disease) can damage the gut and increase its permeability. The luminal contents, which have high concentrations of lipase, can therefore leak out of the gut into the bloodstream, leading to a false-positive elevation in the lipase level. This can lead to a misdiagnosis of pancreatitis, which can result in a missed opportunity for timely surgical intervention in patients with small-bowel obstruction or acute mesenteric ischemia. Clinicians must have a high index of suspicion for other causes of elevated lipase besides acute pancreatitis.

Case 48

A 56-year-old man presents to the gastroenterology clinic complaining of 3 weeks of painful swallowing. All types of food and liquid cause this pain. He does not feel that the food gets stuck and has not vomited. He denies heartburn or recent weight loss.

The patient underwent a liver transplant 3 years ago for cirrhosis secondary to non-alcoholic steatohepatitis. His post-transplant course has been uncomplicated. His other past medical history includes hypertension, dyslipidemia, and diabetes mellitus. His medications include atenolol, simvastatin, insulin glargine, and insulin lispro sliding scale. He also takes immunosuppressive agents (mycophenolate mofetil and tacrolimus) for his liver transplant. He does not smoke or drink alcohol. None of his contacts are unwell and he has not traveled recently.

What is your differential diagnosis?

The differential diagnosis includes reflux esophagitis, infectious esophagitis, esophageal stricture, and esophageal mass.

Physical examination

Vitals Temperature 98.5°F, HR 90 bpm, BP 120/80mmHg, oxygen saturation 99% on RA.

GEN No obvious distress.

HEENT Whitish plaques on the surface of the tongue. Supple neck. No sinus tenderness.

CVS Normal S1, S2. No murmurs, rubs, or gallops.

RESP Clear to auscultation bilaterally.

ABD Prior surgical scar. Soft and non-tender. Bowel sounds are normal.

EXT No edema.

What is the most likely diagnosis, and how will you proceed?

The key point from the history is that the patient is immunocompromised because he has a history of liver transplant. Given his presentation of odynophagia and evidence of whitish plaques on his tongue, the patient probably has Candida esophagitis. However, his immunocompromised status puts him at risk for other bacterial and viral infections.

What imaging test will you order?

In severe cases, a barium esophagram can be diagnostic. For definitive diagnosis, our patient undergoes an EGD (Figure 101).

Describe what you see and read on

This is a photo from the mid-esophagus. It shows whitish plaques that are slightly food-stained. These are easily rubbed off, revealing an inflamed and very friable underlying mucosa.

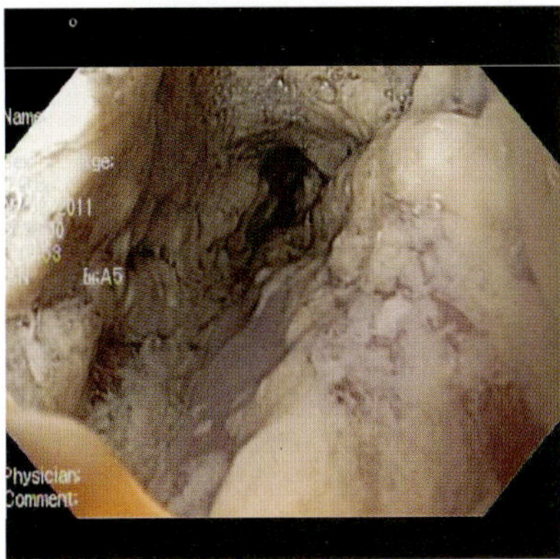

Figure 101.

Biopsies are positive for Candida species and negative for cytomegalovirus or herpes virus. A Gram stain is negative.

What is the next step?

The patient should be started on treatment. Standard therapy consists of a 2-week course of oral fluconazole.

What is a potential problem with antifungal treatment?

Oral antifungal therapy with fluconazole will interact with the patient's metabolism of tacrolimus. He will need frequent monitoring if fluconazole is prescribed. An alternative therapy is oral nystatin (swish and swallow).

Clinical pearls

- In immunocompromised patients with odynophagia and white oral plaques, empiric antifungal therapy can be attempted first; imaging is not always needed. If the patient responds, then the trial is both diagnostic and therapeutic.
- For odynophagia, an EGD is performed in patients with risk factors for Barrett's esophagus (e.g., history of reflux) or esophageal cancer (e.g., smoking, alcoholism, history of Barrett's esophagus), and in those who may have infectious etiologies (e.g., cytomegalovirus, herpes simplex virus, Candida in immunocompromised patients).
- Medication- or pill-induced esophagitis should always be considered in the differential diagnosis. Common culprits include NSAIDs (e.g., naproxen, aspirin, indomethacin, ibuprofen), antibiotics (e.g., tetracycline, doxycycline), procainamide, and bisphosphonates.

Impress your attending

What are the complications of esophagitis?

Complications include strictures, food impaction, bleeding, perforation, and malignancy, as can be seen in reflux esophagitis and Barrett's esophagus.

Case 49

A 61-year-old-man presents to his primary-care physician with a 4-month history of difficulty in swallowing. He initially struggled with solids only, but now finds it difficult to take in liquids as well. He feels a sensation of something "getting stuck" when he swallows. He denies pain on swallowing. He also reports an unintentional weight loss of 20 lbs over the past 6 months.

The patient has a longstanding history of gastroesophageal reflux disease, but this is well controlled with a daily over-the-counter proton-pump inhibitor. His reflux symptoms occur a few times a month. His last EGD was several years ago, and he cannot remember if he had abnormalities or underwent biopsies. He denies vomiting, diarrhea, abdominal pain, hematemesis, or melena. His other past medical history includes controlled hypertension and obesity. The patient has smoked 20 cigarettes daily for the past 30 years. He drinks alcohol only occasionally. There is no family history of GI disease.

Prior to the appointment the primary-care physician ordered routine laboratory tests, including a CBC and basic metabolic profile, which are within normal limits.

What is your differential diagnosis?

The differential diagnosis includes esophageal cancer, Zenker's diverticulum, and esophageal dysmotility, especially achalasia.

Physical examination

Vitals	Temperature 98.3°F, HR 75 bpm, BP 130/70mmHg, oxygen saturation 99% on RA.
GEN	Cachectic appearing.
HEENT	Moist mucous membranes. No scleral icterus. No lymphadenopathy.
CVS	Normal S1, S2. No murmurs, rubs, or gallops.
RESP	Clear to auscultation.
ABD	Abdomen is soft and non-tender. No hepatosplenomegaly. Bowel sounds are normal.
EXT	No clubbing, cyanosis, or edema.

What blood test(s) will you order?

CBC	**WBC**	$6.0 \times 10^3/\mu L$
	Hemoglobin	13.5g/dL
	Hematocrit	39%
	Platelets	$360 \times 10^3/\mu L$
CHEM-7		Normal
LFTs		Normal

Does this narrow your differential diagnosis?

No. The differential diagnosis is unchanged.

Imaging

The patient's primary-care physician orders a barium swallow study and asks the patient to follow

up with a gastroenterologist to discuss the results and any further work-up if indicated.

The barium swallow is shown in Figure 102.

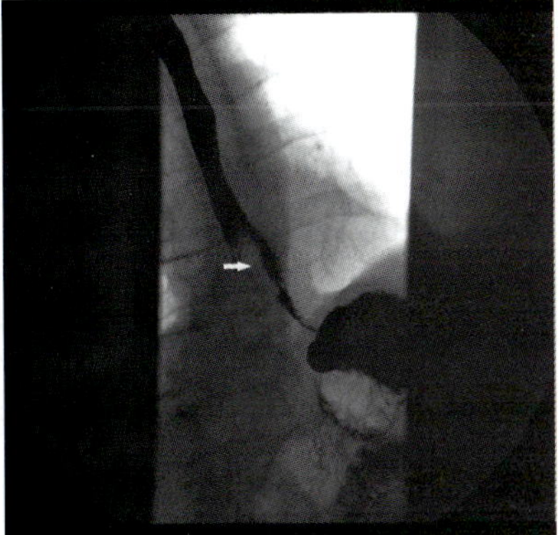

Figure 102.

Describe what you see and read on

This anteroposterior image of the lower esophagus with thin liquid barium shows an irregular, lobulated filling defect (white arrow) causing incomplete obstruction of the distal third of the esophagus. Contrast passes into the fundus of the stomach.

With these results, the gastroenterologist schedules an EGD and endoscopic ultrasound. The patient should be advised to fast overnight prior to the EGD.

The EGD and endoscopic ultrasound images are shown in Figures 103 and 104, respectively.

Describe what you see and read on

The upper endoscopy image (Figure 103) shows an ulcerated and circumferential lesion in the distal esophagus. Biopsies are obtained. Figure 104 shows an endoscopic ultrasound photograph showing the exact location of the mass and its extent in relation to surrounding structures. The mass is anterior to the aorta and abuts but does not invade the wall. There are no enlarged lymph nodes or other masses adjacent to the esophagus.

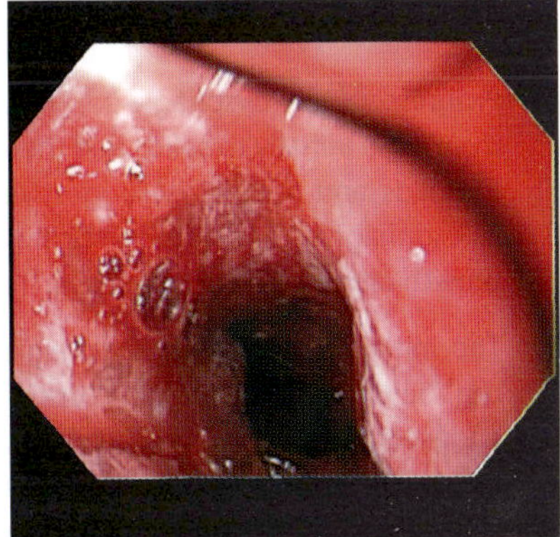

Figure 103.

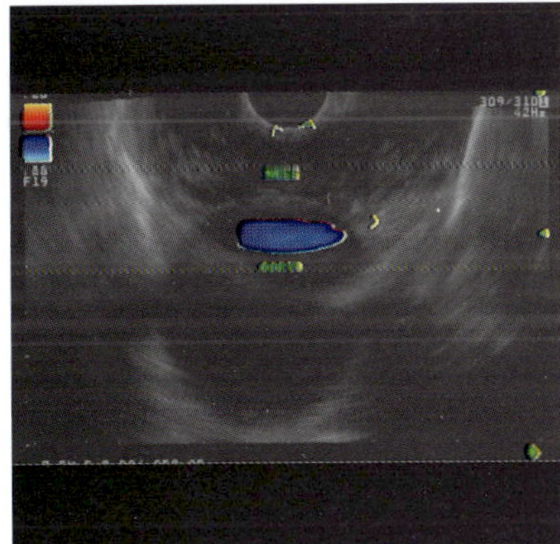

Figure 104.

What is the next step?

The patient has a distal esophageal cancer, and the biopsies confirm esophageal adenocarcinoma. Prior to treatment, a PET CT scan should be obtained of the patient's head through to the mid-thighs to look for metastatic disease. Fortunately for this patient, no other disease was identified.

Given the location and extent of invasion of the adenocarcinoma (through the muscularis and into the periesophageal soft tissues, i.e., T3 staging),

preoperative chemotherapy and radiation are planned prior to distal esophagectomy.

Clinical pearls

- Progressive dysphagia (i.e., dysphagia initially to solids and then to solids and liquids) is suggestive of esophageal cancer and indicates growth or progression of disease.
- The initial evaluation of dysphagia can be conducted with an upper endoscopy or esophagram, depending on availability. Endoscopy is required for tissue diagnosis if a mass is found radiologically.
- Endoscopic ultrasound is employed to assess the local extent of tumor (T) staging. Endoscopic ultrasound with fine-needle aspiration is valuable in assessing the involvement of local lymph nodes, which impacts management.

Impress your attending

What can be a precursor to esophageal adenocarcinoma?

Barrett's metaplasia. This is often caused by longstanding gastroesophageal reflux disease, and needs endoscopic surveillance once identified.

What are other risk factors for the development of esophageal adenocarcinoma?

Smoking and excess alcohol consumption are risk factors for both adenocarcinoma and squamous cell carcinoma of the esophagus. Obesity is an additional risk factor for Barrett's esophagus and adenocarcinoma.

How is esophageal cancer staged?

The TNM staging system is most commonly used:

- T staging refers to tumor size and penetration through the wall of the esophagus. T0 means the primary tumor is undetectable, T1 tumors are confined to the mucosa, T2 masses penetrate through the mucosa into the muscularis propria, T3 lesions penetrate the muscularis into the periesophageal soft tissues, and T4 cancers invade a nearby structure such as the aorta, pleura, pericardium, or diaphragm.
- N staging refers to lymph node involvement. N0 means no nodes detected, N1 signifies nearby lymph node involvement, and N2 indicates the involvement of distant nodes.
- M staging refers to metastatic disease. M0 means no metastases detected, while M1 disease indicates the presence of distant metastases.

For esophageal cancer, the involvement of celiac lymph nodes on endoscopic ultrasound and fine-needle aspiration implies M1 disease, because these nodes are below the diaphragm and are thus considered distant metastases. Endoscopic ultrasound can also occasionally find small liver metastases missed on other imaging studies. This is especially true for the left lobe of the liver, which lies along the lesser curve of the stomach and is well imaged by endoscopic ultrasound.

Case 50

A 64-year-old man presents with acute epigastric pain of 5 hours' duration associated with nausea and vomiting. He denies hematemesis, melena, fever, chills, and weight loss. He is often admitted for pancreatitis caused by alcohol abuse, and was last seen 2 months ago for similar symptoms. At that time, he was managed as an inpatient and was treated with IV fluids, narcotic analgesia, and bowel rest.

The patient had an upper GI bleed 2 years ago caused by erosive gastritis found on endoscopy. He has no other past medical history, but continues to consume large amounts of alcohol each day. He says his symptoms are similar to those of his past episodes of pancreatitis, although he feels his pain is "stronger" this time. The only medication he takes is oxycodone for chronic abdominal pain. He lives alone and is a chronic cigarette smoker.

What is your differential diagnosis?

The differential diagnosis includes acute on chronic pancreatitis, pancreatic pseudocyst, acute alcoholic gastritis, peptic ulcer disease, gastroenteritis, and cholecystitis.

Physical examination

Vitals	Temperature 98.5°F, HR 105 bpm, BP 125/85mmHg, oxygen saturation 98% on RA.
GEN	Appears to be in mild distress.
HEENT	Neck supple. No jugular venous distension. Anicteric.
CVS	Normal S1, S2. No murmurs, rubs, or gallops.
RESP	Clear to auscultation bilaterally.
ABD	Epigastric tenderness. No rebound tenderness or guarding. Bowel sounds are present.
EXT	No edema or bruising.
Skin	No jaundice, spider nevi, or palmar erythema.

What blood test(s) will you order?

CBC	WBC	8.0 x $10^3/\mu L$
	Hemoglobin	12.2g/dL
	Hematocrit	31%
	Platelets	90 x $10^3/\mu L$
	MCV	120mL
CHEM-7		Normal
LFTs	AST	50 units/L
	ALT	30 units/L
	Alkaline phosphatase	250 units/L
	Total bilirubin	1.0mg/dL
Lipase		245 units/L
Amylase		200 units/L

Does this narrow your differential diagnosis?

Yes. The patient has a history of chronic pancreatitis, with a recent episode just 2 months ago. His abdominal pain is now reportedly worse, although he does not have an acute abdomen. His laboratory data reveal evidence of pancreatitis. In addition, he has thrombocytopenia and macrocytic anemia, which are probably a result of alcohol abuse. A low platelet count can also signify cirrhosis.

How will you treat this patient?

The patient is admitted and administered IV fluids and morphine for pain control. He is kept nil by mouth.

What imaging test will you order?

Given worse abdominal pain compared with the patient's baseline, a CT scan of the abdomen should be obtained (Figure 105).

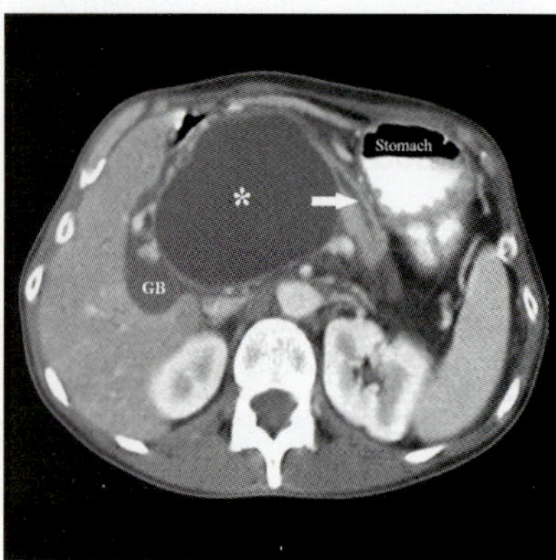

Figure 105.

Describe what you see and read on

An axial CT image with oral and IV contrast through the level of the pancreas is shown. A large pseudocyst (asterisk) is occupying the head of the pancreas adjacent to the gallbladder (GB). The pseudocyst is compressing the duodenum and is also obstructing the pancreatic duct, causing it to dilate (arrow). There is no peripancreatic fat stranding or pancreatic edema to suggest acute pancreatitis.

How do the imaging findings explain the patient's symptoms?

The duodenal compression accounts for the patient's vomiting, while compression of the pancreatic duct accounts for the mild pancreatic enzyme elevations.

The patient underwent transpapillary endoscopic drainage of the pseudocyst by means of a nasal pigtail drain inserted into the pseudocyst cavity through the major papilla. A pancreatic sphincterotomy was also performed. By the third day of admission, the patient's pain had reached his chronic baseline and he was transitioned back to oral pain medications. His lipase level had also reduced significantly and he was tolerating an oral diet. The patient was advised to enroll in an alcohol rehabilitation program.

Clinical pearls

- Pancreatic pseudocysts most commonly occur after recurrent chronic pancreatitis and are a result of pancreatic ductal damage from inflammation. The cysts are lined with a non-epithelialized wall that contains fibrin from chronic inflammation.
- Suspected pancreatic pseudocysts should be investigated to exclude malignancy if the patient has no risk factors for pseudocysts (e.g., a history of pancreatitis) or if the cysts show abnormal features.
- Fluid from pancreatic pseudocysts demonstrates elevated lipase and amylase levels. In malignancy, aspirated fluid is typically low in

lipase and amylase, while the tumor marker carcinoembryonic antigen is often elevated.

Impress your attending

What techniques are available for the drainage and diagnosis of pancreatic and peripancreatic masses?

- Endoscopic ultrasound with transmural (gastric or duodenal) needle puncture with aspiration and stent placement.
- Percutaneous drainage under CT guidance.
- Transpapillary drainage at ERCP by insertion of a stent or nasocystic drain through the major papilla into the main pancreatic duct or even into the cyst itself.
- Surgical drainage, open or laparoscopic.

Look again at the CT image in Figure 105. What finding suggests a higher risk for a surgical approach in this patient?

There is a large, contrast-enhanced gastric varix coursing anteriorly around the pseudocyst and directly beneath the anterior abdominal wall. This is caused by thrombosis of the splenic vein (not shown on this slice), which is a complication of recurrent acute pancreatitis, chronic pancreatitis, and pseudocyst formation.

Other complications of pancreatic pseudocysts include gastric-outlet obstruction with vomiting, biliary obstruction and jaundice, abscesses (infected pseudocysts), and pseudoaneurysm formation with rupture and hemorrhage. The last of these is usually caused by erosion of the pseudocyst into a major artery, typically the splenic artery or superior mesenteric artery.

Index